Contents

Preface to the Second Edition

In 2005, the American College of Sports Medicine published the seventh edition of the *ACSM's Guidelines for Exercise Testing and Prescription*. The new *Guidelines* incorporated several changes that affect how we screen clients and design exercise prescriptions. Risk factor thresholds were modified for fasting glucose, HDL cholesterol, and obesity. New minimal levels of exercise intensity for improving the cardiorespiratory fitness of healthy adults and those with heart disease were recommended. And added emphasis was placed on the importance of higher intensities of exercise for optimizing potential health benefits. Norms for interpreting fitness test results were changed.

The second edition of our book has been thoroughly revised to reflect all of the relevant changes in the ACSM's *Guidelines*. Material has been added to chapter 3 that explains the ACSM's new recommendations for exercise intensity. In fact, these recommendations were based on research that Dr. Swain published with ACSM past-president Barry Franklin. Several chapters have been expanded to provide more information regarding various special populations such as pregnant women, children, and different types of heart patients. All of the material in the case studies has been updated to reflect the ACSM's new screening criteria and new fitness norms. Moreover, the case studies in the appendix have been reformatted to allow easier access to the explanations in the answer section.

Of course, all of the great features of the first edition have been retained, such as the easy reading style and the use of many practical case studies. We trust that this edition will be a valuable tool in expanding your skills in designing exercise prescriptions for a variety of clients, and in preparing for ACSM certification.

Swain, D.P., and B.A. Franklin, 2002. VO_2 Reserve and the minimal intensity for improving cardiorespiratory fitness. *Medicine and Science in Sports and Exercise* 34:152-157.

Swain, D.P., and B.A. Franklin. Is there a threshold intensity for aerobic training in cardiac patients? *Medicine and Science in Sports and Exercise* 34:1071-1075, 2002.

Swain, D.P., and B.A. Franklin. Comparative cardioprotective benefits of vigorous vs. moderate intensity aerobic exercise. *American Journal of Cardiology* 97:141-147, 2006.

1

Case Studies and Risk Stratification

Case studies are an excellent way to learn how to put knowledge into practice. Because case studies provide the learning experience closest to dealing with real-life clients, the American College of Sports Medicine (ACSM) uses them extensively in its certification examinations to illustrate the principles of exercise prescription.

The ACSM's approach to evaluating a case study involves three steps:

1. Screening and risk stratification
2. Assessment of the components of fitness
3. Exercise prescription

This chapter explores the ACSM's basic approach to evaluating case studies, with special attention to screening and risk stratification. Subsequent chapters of this book present case studies that emphasize different elements of this approach. The additional case studies provided in the appendix are comprehensive and challenge you to perform complete evaluations of a variety of real-life clients.

SCREENING AND RISK STRATIFICATION

Renowned exercise physiologist Per-Olaf Åstrand has often said that exercising is safer than remaining sedentary. This is almost universally true, because exercise produces many healthful benefits that reduce the risk of diseases associated with inactivity—coronary heart disease, cerebrovascular disease, type 2 diabetes, osteoporosis, certain forms of cancer, and so on. Yet exercise carries some risk. It increases metabolic demands on the heart and increases sympathetic nervous activity—factors that could trigger a heart attack in people who already have coronary heart disease. Because the many people with undiagnosed heart disease are particularly at risk, screening clients is critical to ensure safety. Before performing exercise testing on clients, and before enrolling them in an exercise program, you should evaluate them to determine their level of risk and to decide whether it is reasonably safe to proceed.

ACSM's Risk Levels

- **Low risk:** Young (44 or younger for men, 54 or younger for women), with no more than one coronary disease risk factor, and without symptoms or known disease
- **Moderate risk:** Older (45 or older for men, 55 or older for women) or with two or more coronary disease risk factors
- **High risk:** With one or more symptoms of cardiopulmonary disease or with known cardiovascular, pulmonary, or metabolic disease (ACSM, 2006)

Table 1.1 provides a screening form for evaluating clients regarding their level of risk to exercise. The form is consistent with the ACSM criteria for risk factor thresholds, symptoms, and relevant known diseases as presented in tables 2-2, 2-3, and 2-4 of the seventh edition of the ACSM *Guidelines*. Unfortunately, the questionnaire presented by the ACSM in that same chapter of the *Guidelines* is *not* consistent with the ACSM's own criteria in its tables 2-2, 2-3, and 2-4. Therefore, we recommend that fitness professionals use the questionnaire presented here. Hopefully, the ACSM will correct its questionnaire in its next edition. One significant discrepancy between the ACSM's criteria and its own questionnaire is that, according to the questionnaire, an older client is placed in the moderate-risk category only if he or she also has at least one additional risk factor. However, according to the ACSM's table 2-4, being older automatically puts the client in the moderate-risk category, even if the client has no other risk factors. Furthermore, the age cutoffs for men and women are one

Table 1.1   Exercise Screening Questionnaire Using ACSM Criteria

Name _____   Sex _____   Date _____

I. Risk Factors (two or more places a person at moderate risk)

_____ 1. Have any of your parents, brothers, or sisters had a heart attack, bypass surgery, angioplasty, or cardiac sudden death? How old was your relative at the time? (Relative must be under 55 if male or under 65 if female to qualify as a risk factor.)

_____ 2. Have you smoked cigarettes in the past six months? (Yes qualifies as a risk factor.)

_____ 3. What is your usual blood pressure? ($\geq$140/90 qualifies as a risk factor.) Do you take blood pressure medication? (Yes qualifies as a risk factor.)

_____ 4. What is your LDL cholesterol level? If you don't know your LDL level, what is your total cholesterol level? What is your HDL cholesterol level? (Either LDL >130 [use total cholesterol >200 if LDL is not known] or HDL <40 qualifies as a risk factor; HDL >60 qualifies as a negative risk factor.)

_____ 5. What is your fasting glucose? ($\geq$100 qualifies as a risk factor.)

_____ 6. What is your height and weight? (BMI $\geq$30 qualifies as a risk factor.) Or ask: What is your waist girth? (Girth of >102 cm, or >40 inches, for a male or >88 cm, or >34.6 inches, for a female qualifies as a risk factor.) Or ask: What are your waist and hip girths? (Waist-to-hip ratio of $\geq$0.95 for a male or $\geq$0.86 for a female qualifies as a risk factor.)

_____ 7. Do you get at least 30 minutes of moderate physical activity most days of the week (or its equivalent)? (No qualifies as a risk factor.)

II. Symptoms (one or more places a person at high risk)

_____ 1. Do you ever have pain or discomfort in your chest or surrounding areas (i.e., ischemia)?

_____ 2. Do you ever feel faint or dizzy (other than when sitting up rapidly)?

_____ 3. Do you find it difficult to breathe when you are lying down or sleeping?

_____ 4. Do your ankles ever become swollen (other than after a long period of standing)?

_____ 5. Do you ever have heart palpitations or an unusual period of rapid heart rate?

(continued)

Table 1.1 *(continued)*

_____ 6. Do you ever experience painful burning or cramping in the muscles of your legs (i.e., intermittent claudication)?

_____ 7. Has a physician ever said that you have a heart murmur? If so, has he or she said it is safe for you to exercise?

_____ 8. Do you feel unusually fatigued or find it difficult to breathe with usual activities?

III. Other

_____ 1. How old are you? (Men ≥45 and women ≥55 are at moderate risk.)

_____ 2. Do you have any of the following diseases: heart disease, peripheral arterial disease, cerebrovascular disease, chronic obstructive pulmonary disease (emphysema or chronic bronchitis), asthma, interstitial lung disease, cystic fibrosis, diabetes mellitus, thyroid disorder, renal disease, or liver disease? (Yes to any disease places the person at high risk.)

_____ 3. Do you have any bone or joint problems, such as arthritis or a past injury, that might get worse with exercise? (If the answer is yes, exercise testing may need to be delayed or modified.)

_____ 4. Do you have a cold or flu, or any other infection? (If yes, exercise testing must be postponed.)

_____ 5. Are you pregnant? (If yes, exercise testing may need to be postponed or modified.)

_____ 6. Do you have any other problem that might make it difficult for you to do strenuous exercise?

▪ *Interpretation*

Low risk (young, and no more than one risk factor): Can do maximal testing or enter a vigorous exercise program.

Moderate risk (older, or two or more risk factors): Can do submaximal testing or enter a moderate exercise program.

High risk (one or more symptoms, or disease): Should not be tested without a physician present; should not begin an exercise program without physician clearance.

Created by the author (DPS) based on information provided in chapter 2 of *ACSM's guidelines for exercise testing and prescription,* 6th edition (ACSM, 2000), and updated with the 7th edition (ACSM, 2006).

year different in the ACSM's questionnaire and its table 2-4. There are other discrepancies as well between the ACSM's questionnaire and the ACSM criteria.

Note that the ACSM screening criteria are intended specifically to determine a client's risk *prior to* exercise and are not intended as a complete list of coronary risk factors. For example, the ACSM is well aware of the fact that exposure to tobacco in any form—chewing tobacco, cigars, pipes, cigarettes, or secondhand smoke—elevates the risk of serious disease. Yet only active cigarette smoking appears in the official criteria, in recognition of the greater risk from this form of exposure. Also note that several risk factor criteria have changed from the sixth to the seventh edition of the ACSM *Guidelines*. Specifically, an HDL cholesterol less than $40 \text{ mg} \cdot dl^{-1}$ is now a risk factor (as opposed to <35), a fasting blood glucose of $100 \text{ mg} \cdot dl^{-1}$ or more is now a risk factor (as opposed to >110), and new criteria have been added for determining the presence of obesity.

When screening clients, always explore the answers to their questions rather than taking simple answers at face value. For example, when asked, "Do you ever have pain or discomfort in your chest or surrounding areas?" a client with a recent muscle strain during bench pressing might answer yes, but would not be at elevated risk of heart disease. Coronary ischemia is not usually experienced as a sharp pain—rather, it appears as a pressure or discomfort, normally occurs during times of stress (including exercise), and is relieved by rest. Similarly, dizziness is common (and benign) when people sit up rapidly. Swelling of the ankles may not indicate cardiovascular complications if it results from long periods of standing with little movement. You must interpret clients' responses with prudent judgment. However, if a client has symptoms that might be due to cardiopulmonary disease, refer him or her to a physician before continuing with exercise testing or programming.

With regards to risk factors, note that each category may be counted only once. For example, if a client's blood pressure is 148/96 mmHg, he or she has an elevated systolic blood pressure and an elevated diastolic blood pressure, but is credited with one risk factor, hypertension. Of course, having *either* an elevated systolic blood pressure *or* an elevated diastolic blood pressure is sufficient to assign the risk factor. Similarly, high LDL and low HDL cholesterol values count singly or together as one risk factor, dyslipidemia.

The interpretation section at the bottom of table 1.1 summarizes the ACSM's recommendations about the form of exercise testing and the intensity of exercise training that clients are ready to enter after the screening process. Low-risk clients are unlikely to experience cardiovascular complications during even the most strenuous exercise. Thus, you can offer low-risk clients submaximal or maximal exercise tests without a physician's supervision, and you can enter these clients into moderate or vigorous exercise programs without first obtaining a physician's clearance.

You can offer moderate-risk clients a submaximal exercise test, such as a bike test performed at a moderate intensity for the prediction of $\dot{V}O_2$max; but you should not give them a maximal exercise test at a health club or other fitness site. Moderate-risk clients should undergo maximal exercise testing only in a clinical setting (i.e., with a physician available in the immediate vicinity). They can enter moderate-intensity exercise programs such as walking clubs or moderate-intensity resistance training but not vigorous programs such as running or competitive sports. If they want to enter a vigorous exercise program, they must first obtain physician clearance—preferably involving a clinically supervised stress test.

High-risk clients should not receive any exercise testing or programming without the direct involvement of the medical community. Exercise tests should be medically supervised. Entry into any exercise program, even of a moderate intensity, needs to be preceded by physician clearance based on stress testing.

CASE STUDY 1.1
Risk Stratification

John is a 42-year-old who is 5'8" (173 cm) tall and weighs 178 lb (80.9 kg). He works as a construction laborer. He has been smoking about a pack of cigarettes per day for over 20 years. His father had a heart attack at age 61. John has no signs or symptoms of cardiopulmonary disease. His blood pressure is 136/82 mmHg on medication. His total cholesterol is 220 mg · dl^{-1}. His fasting glucose is 96 mg · dl^{-1}. He has come to your facility to learn more about ways to reduce his risk of heart disease. How many ACSM risk factors does he have, and what risk stratification category is he in? Can you perform a submaximal or maximal fitness test on him at this time? Can he enter a moderate or vigorous exercise program before obtaining physician clearance?

John has three risk factors: cigarette smoking, hypertension (because he is on medication, even though his current blood pressure is reasonable), and dyslipidemia (based only on knowing his total cholesterol, which is above 200 mg · dl^{-1}). He is not obese, although his body mass index (BMI) of 27.1 kg · m^{-2} puts him in the overweight category (see table 1.2). He would not be classified as sedentary because of his physically active job. He does not have a family history of heart disease *for screening purposes,* because his father's heart attack occurred after the age of 55. His fasting glucose is normal. Although John is considered to be young (under 45), he is in the moderate-risk category because he has at least two risk factors. He is not in the high-risk category because he does not have any signs or symptoms of cardiopulmonary disease or any known cardiovascular, pulmonary, or metabolic disease.

You can safely give John a submaximal test of his cardiovascular fitness as part of an overall appraisal of his condition. He cannot undergo a maximal test unless physician coverage is available. John can safely begin a moderate-intensity exercise program, but he would need physician clearance before embarking on a vigorous exercise program.

Table 1.2   Body Mass Index Categories

BMI (kg · m^{-2})	Category	BMI (kg · m^{-2})	Category
<18.5	Underweight	30.0-34.9	Obesity, class I
18.5-24.9	Normal	35.0-39.9	Obesity, class II
25.0-29.9	Overweight	≥40.0	Obesity, class III (morbid)
≥30.0	ACSM criterion for obesity		

BMI is calculated as body mass in kg divided by the height in meters squared. It may also be calculated from English units as follows: (body weight in lb × 703) / (height in inches squared). The factor 703 converts from English to metric units.

Risk Stratification

Joan is a 32-year-old sales consultant. She smoked three to five cigarettes per day until she quit nine months ago. She is 5'4" (163 cm) tall and weighs 128 lb (58.2 kg). Her grandfather died of heart disease when he was 63. Her mother has type 2 diabetes. Her blood pressure is 106/70 mmHg. She has a total cholesterol level of 192 mg · dl^{-1}, an LDL level of 134 mg · dl^{-1}, and an HDL level of 46 mg · dl^{-1}; her fasting glucose level is 87 mg · dl^{-1}. She walks her dog for 15 to 20 minutes once or twice a day. Stratify Joan's risk status and decide what type of exercise testing and programming she can perform.

Joan has only one risk factor: dyslipidemia. Her total cholesterol is in the desirable range, but LDL cholesterol is more important than total cholesterol. Because her LDL is above the threshold level of 130 mg · dl^{-1}, she meets the criterion for this risk factor. Her HDL is normal, but *either* a high LDL or a low HDL level places a client at risk. Joan has been smoke-free for more than six months, so cigarette smoking is not a risk factor (risk for heart disease drops quickly after smoking cessation, approaching the risk of nonsmokers in one to two years; ex-smokers approach normal risk levels for lung cancer and pulmonary disorders in 10 to 20 years). Joan's BMI is normal at 22.0 kg · m^{-2}. The heart disease in Joan's grandfather and diabetes in her mother do not elevate her own risk of having a heart attack during exercise. Joan would not be considered sedentary because her three hours of walking per week exceeds the ACSM's recommendation of at least two hours of moderate activity per week (i.e., 30 minutes or more on most days of the week; if "most days" is interpreted to mean at least four out of seven, this yields a total of two hours or more per week).

Because Joan has only one risk factor and is young (under 55), she is in the low-risk category. You can give her a maximal test of her aerobic capacity without a physician present. However, you may not need a maximal test: A submaximal test would provide sufficient information to proceed with her exercise prescription. Joan can safely enter a moderate or vigorous exercise program. If you prescribe a vigorous exercise program, be sure to set the initial intensity at a level appropriate for her current level of fitness—not out of fear of a heart attack, but to prevent excessive musculoskeletal strain at the onset of her program.

CASE STUDY 1.3
Risk Stratification

Andy is a 58-year-old public school teacher who is 5'11" (180 cm) tall and weighs 188 lb (85.5 kg). He is a nonsmoker, and his blood pressure is 136/94 mmHg. His brother recently underwent bypass surgery at the age of 52. He plays an hour or more of tennis several afternoons a week and walks 18 holes of golf on Sundays. He complains of pain in the elbow of his dominant arm and of soreness in his ankles. He has no other signs or symptoms, or chronic diseases. His lipid profile is 187 mg · dl^{-1} for total cholesterol, 106 mg · dl^{-1} for LDL, and 68 mg · dl^{-1} for HDL; his fasting glucose level is 96 mg · dl^{-1}. Stratify Andy's risk status and decide what type of exercise testing and programming he can perform.

Andy has two risk factors: hypertension and family history. Because his HDL cholesterol is favorably high, however (above 60 mg · dl^{-1}), you can subtract one risk factor. For screening purposes he therefore has only one risk factor, which would put him in the low-risk category if he were younger. However, because he is over 45, he is automatically placed in the moderate-risk category. Note that hypertension is a risk factor even though only one of the two blood pressure readings, the diastolic in his case, is high. His BMI of 26.2 kg · m^{-2} indicates that he is slightly overweight, but he does not meet the criterion for obesity. His frequent exercise keeps him out of the sedentary category and is the most likely cause of his orthopedic complaints. You can give Andy a submaximal exercise test and prescribe a moderate exercise program at your facility without the need for physician clearance.

CASE STUDY 1.4
Risk Stratification

Alana is a 62-year-old executive in your corporation. During a wellness fair that you provided, the following information was gathered: She is a nonsmoker. She is 5'6" (168 cm) tall, weighs 224 lb (101.8 kg), and has a waist girth of 43" (109 cm). Her blood pressure is 128/84 mmHg, and her lipid profile is as follows: total cholesterol of 218 mg · dl^{-1}, LDL cholesterol of 141 mg · dl^{-1}, HDL cholesterol of 52 mg · dl^{-1}. Her fasting glucose level is 122 mg · dl^{-1}. Her father died

(continued)

Case Study 1.4 *(continued)*

of a heart attack at age 74, and her mother and one of her sisters have type 2 diabetes. Her main form of recreation is reading. She reports no signs or symptoms of chronic diseases. Stratify Alana's risk status and decide what type of exercise testing and programming she can perform.

Alana has three risk factors: obesity, dyslipidemia, and impaired fasting glucose. Obesity is met by two separate criteria—a BMI over 30 kg · m⁻² (hers is 36.2 kg · m⁻²) and a waist girth over 88 cm. Hypercholesterolemia is determined because her LDL reading was over 130 mg · dl⁻¹. Her fasting glucose level is well above the cutoff of 100 mg · dl⁻¹. Note that the fasting glucose test should be repeated to be certain that it is *typically* this high. A fasting glucose >126 mg · dl⁻¹ is the criterion for diagnosing diabetes, but only a physician can make a diagnosis. In a wellness fair, you can only tell her that her fasting glucose is high and that she needs to follow up with her physician.

Technically speaking, Alana is in the moderate-risk category. You can offer her submaximal testing and moderate-intensity exercise programming. However, it would be prudent to wait for her physician's judgment regarding her impaired fasting glucose (i.e., borderline diabetes) before beginning her program.

CASE STUDY 1.5
Risk Stratification

Walter is a 21-year-old college student. He is a varsity track athlete, competing in the shot put and hammer throw. He is 6'1" (185 cm) tall and weighs 245 lb (111.4 kg). His measured body fat is 14%. He is a nonsmoker, and his blood pressure is 128/84 mmHg. His father passed away from a sudden cardiac event at the age of 42. No blood cholesterol or glucose data are available. Walter complains of dizziness when he has to run wind sprints with the track team, and he once passed out briefly after practice. He is being assessed as part of a college wellness class. Stratify his risk.

At first glance, Walter has two risk factors: obesity and family history. Obesity is based on his BMI (32.3 kg · m⁻²) being above the criterion of 30 kg · m⁻². However, because he is a strength athlete, his high BMI may be due simply to his large musculature. This is confirmed by his low body fat measurement; thus he would not be considered obese. More troubling than his risk factors is his complaint of dizziness and syncope during high-intensity exercise. This symptom raises a red flag and automatically places Walter in the high-risk category. He may have a serious congenital abnormality of the heart (which his father may also have had), and it is essential that he be referred to a physician. In fact, you should tell him not to participate in any exercise until he is clinically evaluated.

ASSESSING THE COMPONENTS OF FITNESS

After you screen and stratify clients, your next step is usually to assess their fitness in various areas. Fitness assessment is not mandatory before entering a client into an exercise program, but it is a highly useful step that gives you baseline information to help you design your exercise prescription. It is also useful to repeat assessments at regular intervals to evaluate the client's progress and modify the program. The ACSM emphasizes five components of fitness that have great relevance to health and to functional independence:

1. Body composition (% fat versus % lean body mass; but may also be judged from waist circumference or waist-to-hip ratio or body mass index)
2. Aerobic capacity (maximal aerobic power, $\dot{V}O_2max$)
3. Muscular strength (maximal muscular force, 1RM)
4. Muscular endurance (ability to repeat a given level of contractile force for multiple repetitions)
5. Flexibility (range of motion at a given joint)

You also may want to consider other components of fitness, particularly if athletic performance is at issue. Such additional components would include, but would not be limited to, the following: aerobic endurance, lactate and/or ventilatory thresholds, anaerobic power, anaerobic capacity, reaction time, and balance.

Population norms for the five health-related components of fitness are presented in chapter 4 of the *ACSM's Guidelines for Exercise Testing and Prescription*, seventh edition. These tables will serve as the basis of the fitness interpretations of subsequent case studies, but it is important to recognize that population norms have certain limitations.

One limitation is the population specificity of normative tables. The groups that were tested to provide the norms may not be representative of the types of clients at your facility. For example, some of the ACSM norms are from data collected by the Cooper Institute for Aerobics Research in Dallas. This institution has tested large numbers of clients, thus providing a measure of validity to these norms, but the clients who are able to afford testing at this prestigious institute are hardly representative of average Americans.

Another limitation of norms is that they indicate only what subjects in the test population *were able* to do, not what they *should be able* to do. For example, the "fair" push-up score for women in their 40s is listed as 10 modified (knees on floor) push-ups, whereas the "good" score is listed as 14 modified push-ups. Does this mean that 14 modified push-ups by a 40-something woman is laudatory? Does this truly reflect a high level of muscular fitness, or does it simply reflect low ability in the test group? Because norms are derived from the largely sedentary general population, they may not provide a realistic view of attainable fitness levels, especially in the older cohorts.

A different way to interpret a client's fitness is to employ **criterion standards** (i.e., levels of ability you feel are achievable or desirable) rather than **normative standards.** Our suggestion is that you use population norms (such as those provided by the ACSM) only as a starting point in working with clients. You can later tailor goals to clients' individual abilities and needs.

GOAL SETTING

The most important consideration in setting exercise goals is to include the client in the process. You may have a wealth of information about your clients, such as body composition data, fitness test scores, and lipid values, as well as knowledge about and experience with healthful and prudent goals, but if you simply inform them of their new goals during a consultation, they may not take them to heart. A better strategy is to lead your clients into discovering the goals they should set for themselves. Always maintain a positive and encouraging attitude that helps your clients understand what would be appropriate goals, and be sufficiently open-minded to see when clients are not interested in the goals you believe are appropriate.

Lay out the current situation to the client: "Your aerobic capacity is such-and-such, which for your age and sex is a little below average. More important, it places you at a higher risk for heart disease and means that you can't enjoy many recreational activities." Suggest what would be appropriate and attainable goals: "Fortunately, you can make some real progress in this area with the right exercise program. If you put the effort into it, we could help you to reach the above-average category in just a few months. That would significantly reduce your risk of heart disease and give you the capacity to enjoy an afternoon of tennis without feeling exhausted afterward. On the other hand, a more modest program would at least allow you to reach the average category and help you maintain a reasonable level of fitness for the coming years." At this point you are in a position to ask the client to set the goal: "What would you like to accomplish? Where would you like to be a year from now?"

Following are other important factors to consider in goal setting:

1. Goals should be challenging but attainable.
2. Clients should set long-term and short-term goals.
3. Goals should be highly specific and practical.
4. Clients should enlist social support to help them reach their goals.

Goals should be challenging but attainable. Don't fall into the pattern of expecting little progress from a client just because in your experience many clients don't make dramatic improvements. Dramatic improvements are indeed possible, and you need to project confidence that the client can make great changes. Ask clients to think about how they would really like to be a year or two from now. Lose 100 lb (45 kg) and look fit and trim? Lower total cholesterol from 300 to well under 200 mg · dl^{-1}? Improve aerobic capacity from couch potato status to marathon finisher? All of these are very achievable for most people. Give your clients the motivation to reach for their dreams. However, changes like these do not happen overnight. If a client announces, "I've never run before and I want to run a marathon next month," your response can be, "Great, but let's aim for next year." Some clients may have unrealistic goals. To a client who says, "I want to be national champion in my sport someday," you can respond, "You've been competing in your sport for several years and are still at a regional level; we can help you improve, but your aerobic power [or muscle strength or whatever] isn't likely to reach elite levels."

Lofty goals for the future are admirable, provided they are also realistic, but what will the client accomplish in the next week or month? Help clients break down long-term goals into short-term, manageable segments. This provides a framework for setting workout plans and evaluating progress. It also provides frequent reinforcement as clients attain intermediate goals. A desire to lose 100 lb (45 kg) in the next two years can be lost if the person sees no progress in the next two weeks.

Goals to improve fitness, lower cholesterol, or lose weight are appropriate as a starting point. But such general goals are not meaningful in a practical sense. Goals must be translated into a highly specific, personalized plan of action. Consider a goal to lower cholesterol by 50 points through a decrease in dietary fat intake. What specific new foods is the client committing to eating? Drinking skim milk instead of whole milk, eating fish instead of red meat, and using olive oil instead of saturated and hydrogenated fats? The client needs goals associated with adopting new behaviors, not just numbers from a blood test. Or consider a goal to improve aerobic capacity from the average to the above-average category. This goal needs to be expressed in terms of behavior change, in association with a detailed exercise prescription. For example, the client may commit to walking briskly for 20 to 30 minutes four times a week. When, exactly, will she do this walking? Ask her to verbalize the days of the week and the times of day she will walk. Write it down as part of the exercise prescription. Of course, some flexibility is needed in putting these changes into action, but obtaining a clear commitment from the client *for specific behaviors,* and not just outcomes, makes the goal more concrete and more likely to be accomplished.

Social support is a key element to successful behavior change. Humans are social animals, and much of human behavior is based on seeking the approval of others. If family members or coworkers scoff at clients' new behaviors, it will be much harder for them to achieve their goals. Try to turn clients' desire for approval to their advantage: Involve family members in the program; run team contests at work sites; enlist partners in a buddy system; and target highly visible and respected people for programming, such as company CEOs. Tapping into the power of social support is an important ingredient in helping clients to achieve their goals.

EXERCISE PRESCRIPTION

After clients are screened and their goals are established, exercise prescription is the next step. Keep in mind, however, that writing exercise prescriptions and establishing goals are interrelated tasks. It is not practical to design a fully developed exercise prescription without knowing a client's goals, but some basic principles of exercise prescription apply to most situations. Chapter 2 discusses these principles, and table 2.1 summarizes the associated ACSM guidelines.

To be certified as an ACSM Health/Fitness Instructor, you must be able to apply these general guidelines. To work with clients in day-to-day practical situations, you should be able to master the details of these guidelines to set specific exercise prescriptions that are tailored to the needs of individual clients. Subsequent chapters will explore these guidelines for exercise prescription in more detail.

REFERENCES

ACSM. 2006. *ACSM's Guidelines for Exercise Testing and Prescription*, 7th ed., 21-28. Philadelphia: Lippincott Williams & Wilkins. Expert Panel. 1998. Executive summary of the clinical guidelines on the identification, evaluation, and treatment of overweight and obesity in adults. *Archives of Internal Medicine* 158: 1855-1867.

Expert Panel. 1998. Executive summary of the clinical guidelines on the identification, evaluation, and treatment of overweight and obesity in adults. *Archives of Internal Medicine* 158: 1855-1867.

2

Basic Principles
for Exercise Prescription,
Now With V̇O₂ Reserve

The principles for prescribing exercise have been developed over centuries of human activity and athletic conditioning and refined over the past few decades of scientific research. This chapter presents an overview of these principles and introduces the American College of Sports Medicine (ACSM) guidelines for exercise prescription that will be followed throughout this book.

PRINCIPLES OF TRAINING

Living organisms adapt to stress. This basic aspect of all life is the foundation of exercise training. When people increase their effort a little more than normal (called an "overload" by exercise physiologists), their bodies respond by improving strength, flexibility, aerobic capacity, or any other component of fitness that the activity challenged. Although any form of overload induces a response, to get the best results one needs to perform the exercise in a well-designed, systematic fashion.

Years of research have uncovered several guiding principles for optimum exercise training. Of special note are the principles of overload, adaptation, progression, specificity, recovery, overtraining, detraining, and individual responsiveness.

Overload and Adaptation

In figure 2.1, the vertical axis presents the maximum capacity of a system. This capacity could refer to aerobic power (i.e., maximal oxygen consumption, or $\dot{V}O_2max$), muscular strength (i.e., one repetition maximum, or 1RM), or some other capacity. Each bout of exercise—when performed as an **overload**—initially results in fatigue and a temporary decrease in capacity. As the system recovers from the bout of exercise, the capacity increases to a level greater than the original value (see figure 2.1*a*). This increase is due to a number of physiological **adaptations** that are inherent to living things. For a partial list of these adaptations, see "Adaptations to Aerobic Training" on page 20 and "Adaptations to Resistance

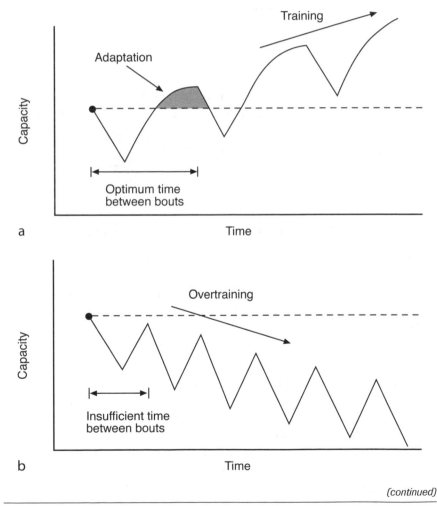

a

b

(continued)

Figure 2.1   Illustration of the adaptive response of training. In 2.1*a*, the proper spacing of exercise bouts allows full recovery and adaptation, resulting in *training*. In 2.1*b*, bouts are spaced too close together, preventing full recovery and resulting in *overtraining*.

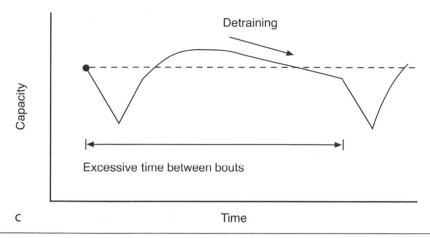

Capacity

Detraining

Excessive time between bouts

c

Time

Figure 2.1 (*continued*) In 2.1*c*, bouts are spaced too far apart, resulting in a loss of adaptation and *detraining*.

Training" on page 21. Most of these changes are typically too small to be measured after a single bout of exercise, but their cumulative effect over many bouts of exercise is referred to as training.

Progression

The principle of **progression** states that *the exercise stimulus must increase over time in order to elicit continued improvements*. For example, lifting a 10 lb (4.5 kg) dumbbell in a biceps curl might increase a person's strength; but if that person stays with that weight for several weeks, the strength will increase only in the first week or two but will not improve after that point. The intensity, duration, or frequency of the stimulus must gradually increase for gains in strength to continue. A popular variation of this principle is periodization, in which the stimulus varies in a structured pattern over time, including periods of relative recovery—yet the overall effect is that the stimulus increases.

Specificity

It is important to recognize that the adaptations induced by training are highly **specific** to the stress. One obvious example is that resistance training increases strength but has a minimal effect on aerobic capacity. Furthermore, the increased strength arises in the muscles that were exercised but not in other muscles (although a small amount of crossover improvement can be observed in the

Adaptations to Aerobic Training

- Increased parasympathetic tone/decreased sympathetic tone— reduced HR at rest and during submaximal exercise, slightly reduced maximal HR

- Increased size of the left ventricle (proportional increase in wall thickness and chamber diameter, eccentric hypertrophy)— increased stroke volume at rest and during both submaximal and maximal exercise

- Increased cardiac output, workload, and oxygen consumption at maximal exercise

- Increased plasma volume

- Increased maximal ventilation, decreased ventilation during submaximal exercise (improved economy of breathing)

- Decreased resistance to blood flow in trained muscles—reduced BP at rest and during submaximal exercise

- Increased number of capillaries—reduced diffusion distance for oxygen

- Increased myoglobin in muscle cells—increased oxygen transport to mitochondria

- Substantial increase in mitochondria and associated enzymes

- Increased use of fat—glycogen-sparing, increased endurance at submaximal workload

- Increased insulin sensitivity

- Increased lactate removal by organs—increased lactate threshold, tolerance of high-intensity effort

- Increased ATP (adenosine triphosphate), CP (creatine phosphate), and glycogen stores

muscles of the opposite limb when only one limb is trained, as a result of neural adaptations). These examples are obvious, but they illustrate a principle that is present in more subtle applications. For example, resistance training on an isokinetic machine (which varies the resistance to produce a constant angular speed of movement at a joint) results in large increases in strength *on that device*. But when the isokinetically trained muscles perform

Adaptations to Resistance Training

- Increased motor unit recruitment—ability to simultaneously contract a greater percentage of motor units resulting in increased strength
- Increased growth of myofilaments—muscle cell hypertrophy, and thus muscle hypertrophy resulting in increased strength
- Possible long-term conversion of Type I to Type II fibers
- Possible proliferation of muscle cells (hyperplasia)—muscle hypertrophy
- Increased stores of ATP, CP, and glycogen
- Increased left ventricular size (wall thickness more than chamber diameter, concentric hypertrophy)

similar movements using standard machines or free weights (that have a constant external load), they will exhibit much smaller increases in strength. The reason for this effect is that *most of the strength increase after resistance training is due to improved **neural recruitment patterns,*** which are specific to the way the muscle is asked to contract. Only a small portion of the strength improvement is due to muscle hypertrophy, which is generalized to any activity performed by the muscle. An example of specificity from aerobic training is that very little of the improvement in aerobic capacity after one mode of training (e.g., running) is evident when the person performs a different mode of exercise that uses many of the same muscle groups (e.g., cycling).

Recovery, Overtraining, Detraining

In figure 2.1, the horizontal axis presents time. The distance between bouts of exercise is the **recovery** time. Workouts must be spaced carefully to obtain the best results. The body needs time to recover and replenish energy stores and for adaptive processes to take place. The length of recovery time needed between bouts varies directly with the overall stress (both the intensity and volume) of the exercise session. Obviously, highly intense or lengthy bouts of exercise require greater recovery times than less intense or shorter bouts. If the bouts are spaced too closely together, insufficient recovery will take place before the next session occurs, leading to **overtraining** (see figure 2.1*b*); if too much time occurs between bouts, the adaptation will be lost and **detraining** will occur (see figure 2.1*c*).

The optimum spacing of workouts depends on numerous interdependent factors, chief among them being the overall stress of the workout; the type of exercise being performed (e.g., resistive, aerobic, flexibility); and the person's current training status, fitness level, and nutritional status. People typically perform resistance training only once every two or three days, but the schedule varies with the intensity of the workout. During rehabilitation from an injury, resistance training may occur as often as twice per day but with very low resistance. Alternatively, some weightlifting athletes may train a given muscle group as infrequently as once a week, to provide sufficient recovery from extremely intense exercise. Aerobic training is generally performed at least three times per week but can be done daily or even twice daily in both rehabilitation and athletic conditioning. Endurance athletes must build up to high training frequencies (and durations) over extended periods of time, and they must pay special attention to nutritional needs (primarily a high carbohydrate intake to replenish glycogen stores), orthopedic tolerance, and signs of overtraining. Flexibility training is best done on a daily or twice-daily basis, but less frequent training can still yield meaningful results.

Individual Responsiveness

The adaptive responses of the human body to various exercise regimens are well known and allow exercise professionals to develop exercise prescriptions and workout routines that can be widely applied to the general population. However, individual responses to training will vary. Some clients improve more quickly than others do. As discussed earlier, recovery time between workouts can vary considerably as a result of many individual factors. Furthermore, many clients may have orthopedic conditions or health problems, or may be taking a variety of medications, that require special consideration in exercise prescription. For these reasons, you must consider national guidelines, such as those of the ACSM, as a starting point in working with clients. Always be prepared to adjust workloads up or down based on the immediate responses of a client to an exercise session, as well as on the overall progress that the client is making over time.

ACSM GUIDELINES

The ACSM has taken a leading role in the study of exercise physiology and the practice of exercise prescription. Its recommendations have been published since the first edition of *Guidelines for Graded Exercise Testing and Exercise Prescription* in 1975 (ACSM, 1975), and they have been systematically reviewed and refined in succeeding editions. In 1998 the ACSM published a landmark position stand in its scientific journal, *Medicine and Science in Sports and Exercise*, on "The Recommended Quantity and Quality of Exercise for Developing and Maintaining Cardiorespiratory and Muscular Fitness, and Flexibility in Healthy Adults" (Pollock et al., 1998). This position stand synthesized a vast body of knowledge about the scientific aspects of exercise training and put forth recommendations for exercise prescription. In 2006 the most recent refinement of these recommendations was published in the seventh edition of *ACSM's Guidelines for Exercise Testing and Prescription*, the "bible" of exercise professionals.

Table 2.1 summarizes the ACSM's current recommendations for cardiovascular, muscular strength, and flexibility training (ACSM, 2006). These recommendations are intended to provide a framework for exercise professionals who work with the general population, as opposed to the opposite extremes of patients and athletes. However,

Table 2.1 ACSM Exercise Prescription Principles

Category	Frequency	Intensity	Time	Type
Cardiovascular	Three to five days per week	40/50-85% of HRR or $\dot{V}O_2R$	20-60 min	Large muscle mass, continuous, rhythmic
Muscular strength	Two or three days per week	3- to 20RM range, typically 8- to 12RM	One set each of 8-10 exercises ($\leq$1 hr)	Major muscle groups, full ROM, controlled speed (~3 s concentric, ~3 s eccentric)
Flexibility	Two or three days per week, ideally five to seven	To point of tightness	15-30 s for each of two to four reps	Static

Created by the author (DPS) based on information provided in chapter 7 of *ACSM's guidelines for exercise testing and prescription,* 6th edition (ACSM, 2000), and updated with the 7th edition (ACSM, 2006).

as later chapters will explore, the basic principles require only modest modifications when working with these specialized groups. These guidelines follow the **FITT principle,** in which F stands for frequency of exercise (days per week), I stands for intensity (% of maximum capacity), T stands for time (duration on a given day), and T stands for type (the mode of exercise).

In tables 2.1 and 2.2, the term HRR stands for **heart rate reserve** (i.e., a percentage of the difference between resting and maximal HR). The term $\dot{V}O_2R$ refers to **$\dot{V}O_2$ reserve,** which is similarly defined as a percentage of the difference between resting and maximal $\dot{V}O_2$. Intensity for resistance training is indicated as "8- to 12RM," which means the range from the 8-repetition maximum to the 12-repetition maximum. The 8RM is a weight that can be lifted eight times in succession but not nine times. Such a weight is approximately 84% of a person's 1RM. Similarly, a 12RM load is a weight that can be lifted 12 but not 13 times and is approximately 76% of 1RM. The term ROM stands for **range of motion.** The specific information presented in table 2.2 will be examined in much more detail in the succeeding chapters and applied to a variety of practical case studies.

Table 2.2   Equivalent Exercise Intensities Using %HRR, %$\dot{V}O_2R$, and %$\dot{V}O_2$max

%HRR	%$\dot{V}O_2R$	%$\dot{V}O_2$max		
		5 MET capacity	10 MET capacity	20 MET capacity
0% (rest)	0%	20%	10%	5%
40%	40%	52%	46%	43%
50%	50%	60%	55%	53%
85%	85%	88%	87%	86%
100%	100%	100%	100%	100%

%HRR units and %$\dot{V}O_2R$ units provide equivalent intensities throughout the range from rest to maximal exercise (e.g., if a client is at 50% of heart rate reserve, he or she is also at 50% of $\dot{V}O_2$ reserve). Units of %$\dot{V}O_2$max must be adjusted to achieve the same intensity. Furthermore, the amount of adjustment needed in the %$\dot{V}O_2$max units varies with the fitness level of the client. The table illustrates this principle for three different clients, one with a 5 MET capacity (deconditioned), one with a 10 MET capacity (average sedentary adult), and one with a 20 MET capacity (endurance athlete).

$\dot{V}O_2$ RESERVE

The use of $\dot{V}O_2$ reserve was first adopted by the ACSM in its 1998 position stand. Previously, the ACSM recommended that exercise prescriptions for cardiorespiratory fitness be based on a percentage of $\dot{V}O_2$max. It had been assumed that clients could achieve a given percentage of $\dot{V}O_2$max by having them exercise at that same percentage of heart rate reserve (HRR). That is, if one wished a client to exercise at 60% of $\dot{V}O_2$max, the target HR would be calculated at 60% of HRR (take 60% of the difference between HRmax and HRrest, and then add this product to HRrest).

However, research by the authors of this book demonstrated that there is an error between %HRR and %$\dot{V}O_2$max (Swain and Leutholtz, 1997; Swain et al., 1998). This error is easiest to observe at rest. When a person is resting, he or she is by definition at 0% of HRR (0% of a *range* is simply the low end of the range) but is not at 0% of $\dot{V}O_2$max, because that would be a $\dot{V}O_2$ of 0. The person would have to be dead, not resting, to be at 0% of $\dot{V}O_2$max! As figure 2.2 shows, the error between %HRR and %$\dot{V}O_2$max *at rest* can be quite large, depending on the client's fitness level. A typical person has a $\dot{V}O_2$ at rest of 3.5 ml $\cdot$ min^{-1} $\cdot$ kg^{-1} (or 1 MET) and a $\dot{V}O_2$max that is 10 times higher, or 35 ml $\cdot$ min^{-1} $\cdot$ kg^{-1} (i.e., 10 METs). This person would therefore be at 1/10 of $\dot{V}O_2$max, or 10%, when resting. A poorly fit client, with a maximal capacity of only 17.5 ml $\cdot$ min^{-1} $\cdot$ kg^{-1}, or 5 METs, would be at 1/5, or 20% of $\dot{V}O_2$max at rest. On the other hand, there is very little error between %HRR and %$\dot{V}O_2$max for highly fit clients, as illustrated in figure 2.2 by the person with a 20 MET capacity (70 ml $\cdot$ min^{-1} $\cdot$ kg^{-1}) who is at 1/20, or 5%, of $\dot{V}O_2$max when resting.

The error between %HRR and %$\dot{V}O_2$max becomes gradually smaller as exercise intensity increases, because both %HRR and %$\dot{V}O_2$max are approaching 100%. The error is most noticeable in clients with a low fitness level who are exercising at a low intensity. In research by the current authors, we introduced the term *$\dot{V}O_2$ reserve ($\dot{V}O_2R$)* to represent the percentage of the difference between resting and maximal $\dot{V}O_2$. Of course, when a person is resting, he or she is at 0% of HRR and also 0% of $\dot{V}O_2$R. Consequently, we demonstrated that there is no error between these terms throughout the range of exercise intensities, from rest up to maximum

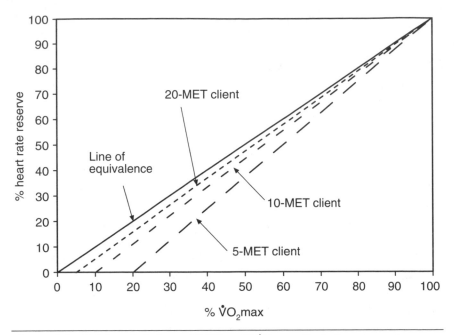

Figure 2.2 Relationship between %HRR and %$\dot{V}O_2$max, illustrating a large discrepancy between these two indicators of intensity, especially at lower levels of exercise (i.e., the distance between the clients' lines and the line of equivalence). This discrepancy between %HRR units and %$\dot{V}O_2$max units is larger for clients with lower fitness levels, as seen by the greater distance from the line of equivalence for the 5 MET client compared to the 10 MET and 20 MET clients.

(see figure 2.3). That is to say, a client can be placed at any desired percentage of $\dot{V}O_2$R by using that same percentage of HRR: 40% of HRR is equivalent to 40% of $\dot{V}O_2$R, 60% of HRR is equivalent to 60% of $\dot{V}O_2$R, and so on. Table 2.2 provides the values of %HRR, %$\dot{V}O_2$R, and %$\dot{V}O_2$max at equivalent levels of exercise intensity. Values of %$\dot{V}O_2$max are presented for three people with different fitness levels. Fitness level does not affect the values for %HRR and %$\dot{V}O_2$R, because all clients are placed at similar levels of intensity *relative to their own ability* by using these terms. Use the following formula to calculate a target intensity using $\dot{V}O_2$R:

$\dot{V}O_2$ Reserve Formula:

Target $\dot{V}O_2$ = (intensity fraction)($\dot{V}O_2$max − $\dot{V}O_2$rest) + $\dot{V}O_2$rest

Since resting $\dot{V}O_2$ averages 3.5 ml · min^{-1} · kg^{-1}, this can be rewritten as

Target $\dot{V}O_2$ = (intensity fraction)($\dot{V}O_2$max − 3.5) + 3.5

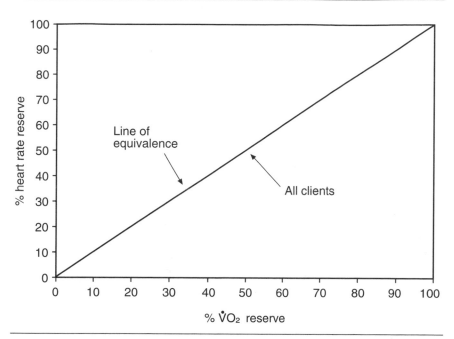

Figure 2.3   In contrast to figure 2.2, the relationship between %HRR and %$\dot{V}O_2$ reserve falls along the line of equivalence (i.e., %HRR units and %$\dot{V}O_2$R units provide equivalent indicators of exercise intensity).This is true for clients of all fitness levels, making %$\dot{V}O_2$R very useful for exercise prescription.

Our research used young, healthy adults exercising on both cycle ergometers and treadmills. After its publication, the ACSM adopted the use of $\dot{V}O_2$R for establishing intensity in exercise prescriptions in its position stand (Pollock et al., 1998) and in its *Guidelines* (ACSM, 2000, 2006). Since that time, other researchers have confirmed the relationship between %HRR and %$\dot{V}O_2$R—in older, healthy adults (Down and Haennel, 1997), in cardiac patients with or without beta-blocker medication (Brawner et al., 2002), and in diabetic patients with or without autonomic neuropathy (Colberg et al., 2003). The following case study illustrates the effect of using %$\dot{V}O_2$R in exercise prescriptions.

C A S E   S T U D Y   2 . 1
Use of %$\dot{V}O_2$R vs. %$\dot{V}O_2$max in an Exercise Prescription

Susan is a 57-year-old woman who is very deconditioned. She is 5'5" tall (165 cm) and weighs 187 lb (85 kg). Her body mass index (BMI) is 31 kg · m⁻², which places her in the class I obesity category.

(continued)

Case Study 2.1   *(continued)*

She is sedentary, has a family history of heart disease, and has an elevated resting blood pressure (146/92 mmHg). Because she recently complained of shortness of breath, her physician ordered a stress test. She performed the modified Bruce protocol and completed stage I (1.7 mph or 2.7 kph, 10% grade) with a maximal HR of 158 bpm and no indications of coronary ischemia. Her aerobic capacity was estimated from the treadmill protocol as 5 METs (i.e., 17.5 ml · min^{-1} · kg^{-1}). What is an appropriate exercise prescription to improve her aerobic conditioning?

At this point we will not examine a detailed treatment of Susan's current condition and exercise prescription—only the issue of how the use of %$\dot{V}O_2R$ versus %$\dot{V}O_2$max affects the prescription. Because of her poor fitness status, you should set her initial exercise intensity at a low level. According to table 2.2, the ACSM recommends that a prescription can begin as low as 40% of $\dot{V}O_2R$. You decide that her target $\dot{V}O_2$ during exercise will be as follows:

$$\text{Target } \dot{V}O_2 = (\text{intensity fraction})(\dot{V}O_2\text{max} - 3.5) + 3.5$$

$$= 0.40(17.5 - 3.5) + 3.5$$

$$= 0.40(14) + 3.5$$

$$= 5.6 + 3.5$$

$$= 9.1 \text{ ml · min}^{-1} \cdot \text{kg}^{-1}$$

As chapter 4 will explain, the ACSM's metabolic equations can translate a target $\dot{V}O_2$ into a workload on a piece of exercise equipment. In this case, 9.1 ml · min^{-1} · kg^{-1} yields a treadmill walking speed of 2.1 mph (3.4 kph). If 40% of $\dot{V}O_2$max had been used instead of 40% of $\dot{V}O_2R$, the target $\dot{V}O_2$ would have been only 0.40 × 17.5 = 7 ml · min^{-1} · kg^{-1}, which translates to a walking speed of 1.3 mph (2.1 kph). Thus, the use of %$\dot{V}O_2$max would have placed her at a walking speed that is almost 40% less than she actually needs. Furthermore, if you use a target HR to determine her exercise intensity, you need to recognize that 40% of HRR would result in the higher of these two walking speeds.

In case study 2.1, %$\dot{V}O_2$max introduced a large error in the prescribed exercise intensity, relative to the client's ability. As mentioned earlier, the error would be smaller for more fit clients or for clients exercising at higher percentages of their capacity. The use of $\%\dot{V}O_2max$ in exercise prescriptions for endurance athletes introduces only minimal errors. Nevertheless, for the sake of consistency, this book will follow the ACSM's recommendation of using $\%\dot{V}O_2R$ instead of $\%\dot{V}O_2max$ whenever there is a need to establish an exercise intensity from $\dot{V}O_2$.

REFERENCES

ACSM. 1975. *Guidelines for Graded Exercise Testing and Exercise Prescription.* Philadelphia: Lea & Febiger.

ACSM. 2000. *ACSM's Guidelines for Exercise Testing and Prescription*, 6th ed., 137-164. Philadelphia: Lippincott Williams & Wilkins.

ACSM. 2006. *ACSM's Guidelines for Exercise Testing and Prescription*, 7th ed., 133-173. Philadelphia: Lippincott Williams & Wilkins.

Brawner, C.A., S.J. Keteyian, and J.K. Ehrman. 2002. The relationship of heart rate reserve to $\dot{V}O_2$ reserve in patients with heart disease. *Medicine and Science in Sports and Exercise* 34: 418-422.

Colberg, S.R., D.P. Swain, and A. Vinik. 2003. Use of heart rate reserve and rating of perceived exertion to prescribe exercise intensity in diabetic autonomic neuropathy. *Diabetes Care* 26: 986-990.

Down, R.J., and R.G. Haennel. 1997. Percent heart rate reserve is not equivalent to percent maximal oxygen uptake (abstract). *Canadian Journal of Applied Physiology* 22 (Suppl.): 13P.

Pollock, M.L., G.A. Gaesser, J.D. Butcher, J.P. Despres, R.K. Dishman, B.A. Franklin, and C.E. Garber. 1998. The recommended quantity and quality of exercise for developing and maintaining cardiorespiratory and muscular fitness, and flexibility in healthy adults (ACSM position stand). *Medicine and Science in Sports and Exercise* 30: 975-991.

Swain, D.P., and B.C. Leutholtz. 1997. Heart rate reserve is equivalent to $\%\dot{V}O_2$Reserve, not to $\%\dot{V}O_2max$. *Medicine and Science in Sports and Exercise* 29: 410-414.

Swain D.P., B.C. Leutholtz, M.E. King, L.A. Haas, and J.D. Branch.1998. Relationship of % heart rate reserve and % $\dot{V}O_2$Reserve in treadmill exercise. *Medicine and Science in Sports and Exercise* 30: 318-321.

3

Exercise Prescription for Cardiorespiratory Fitness

As noted in chapter 2 and summarized in table 2.1, cardiorespiratory exercise prescriptions are based on the FITT principle: frequency, intensity, time (duration), and type (mode). This chapter briefly examines type, frequency, and time, and then explains in detail the ACSM's recommendations for prescribing intensity.

TYPE (MODE)

A cardiorespiratory exercise is one that stimulates a substantial, sustained increase in oxygen consumption. To do this, the exercise must use a large amount of muscle mass. Thus, although operating a rowing machine with just the arms is aerobic, it is not as effective for cardiorespiratory training as performing the exercise with the arms, legs, and back. To obtain a sustained increase in oxygen consumption, the exercise must be continuous and rhythmic: Repetitive activities such as walking, running, rowing, bicycling, and swimming are more aerobic than stop-and-go sports such as tennis and basketball.

FREQUENCY AND TIME (DURATION)

The recommended frequency of cardiorespiratory exercise is three to five days per week, with a duration of 20 to 60 minutes per day (ACSM, 2006). Most clients just starting an exercise program are able to begin with three times a week for 20 minutes. Depending on their goals, they should then progress toward the upper range of frequency and duration (possibly increasing intensity as well).

Progression should occur gradually and be tailored to individual responsiveness to the training program. A prudent goal for many clients would be to increase the total volume of exercise by 10% per week.

The exercise time can be accumulated over two or more sessions in a day to achieve the desired total, although one cannot simply add up various daily chores and call this a training program. Sixty 1-minute trips to the water fountain do not add up to an hour of aerobic exercise! Each exercise session needs to be a distinct period of time in which the proper intensity is maintained, not including the warm-up and cool-down.

Both warm-ups and cool-downs should entail 5 to 10 minutes of low-intensity exercise that emphasizes the same muscles used in the exercise session. The warm-up period increases the temperature and elasticity of the muscles and elicits increases in breathing, heart action, and muscle blood flow that prepare the body for the more vigorous exercise to come. The cool-down prevents blood pooling by maintaining the "muscle pump" effect in which the active muscles massage their own veins to help propel blood toward the heart. The cool-down also helps clear lactic acid from the bloodstream.

Flexibility training is best done at the end of the cool-down when the muscles are still warm and elastic. Clients who like to do stretching before they exercise should be instructed to delay the stretching at least until after they have completed their warm-up.

A frequency of fewer than three days per week may not be sufficient for improving cardiorespiratory fitness, although it may allow for maintenance of a moderate fitness level. A frequency of more than five days per week will provide diminishing returns of improvement for the amount of time and effort expended, and it may lead to overtraining or orthopedic problems. Yet most people, if they increase their schedule quite gradually, can successfully perform cardiorespiratory exercise on a daily basis. People who exercise three or four times per week should do so on alternate days, to allow their bodies maximum recovery time between sessions.

The ACSM recommends that the duration of 20 to 60 minutes should be used in a complementary manner with intensity. To burn a given number of calories, people can exercise at a high intensity for a short period of time, or at a low intensity for a long period of time. In practice, most fit clients exercise with a longer duration *and* a higher intensity than less fit clients, but the ACSM recommendations aim to develop a desirable level of health-related fitness for the general population.

CASE STUDY 3.1
Cardiorespiratory Exercise Prescription

Yolanda is a 33-year-old moderate-risk client. She is overweight and sedentary but otherwise appears healthy. She states that she would like to become more fit, but she has trouble finding time in her schedule for exercise. Design a general exercise program for her to improve cardiorespiratory fitness.

Ask Yolanda if there are any types of aerobic exercise that she enjoyed when she was younger, or that she enjoys watching other people perform. Help her select a mode of exercise that is fun and that entails little initial equipment or expense. For many clients, walking is a great choice. If she tries one mode of exercise for a couple of weeks and doesn't like it, help her to choose another. Explain to her that exercise is critical to health, and that she should make an initial commitment to perform 20 minutes of exercise, three times a week, at a moderate intensity. (The initial intensity should be 50% of $\dot{V}O_2R$; prescribing intensity will be explained in more detail later in this chapter.) Help her to find a specific time, or times, in her day when she is doing things that are of lower priority. (To make time for exercise, some people choose to watch less television in the evenings, to go to bed a little earlier and then exercise in the morning, or to schedule an exercise break during the workday. Without health, all other pursuits in life are unattainable. Thus, most activities earn a lower priority than regular exercise.) Be sure also to teach Yolanda how to warm up and cool down.

Next, discuss exercise progression with Yolanda. Although she is starting with 20 minutes, three times a week, she will want to gradually increase her exercise duration to achieve the best results. For example, each week she could add five minutes to each exercise session, until she reaches perhaps an hour. She could divide the hour into two or three sessions per day if that helps her achieve her duration goal. And she could add one day every other week until she is working out five days per week. She could also increase

(continued)

Case Study 3.1   *(continued)*

the intensity gradually so that the workout remains challenging while still being enjoyable (not to exceed the ACSM upper limit of 85% $\dot{V}O_2R$). You can reevaluate her in one or two months, and every few months thereafter, adjusting the program to best meet her goals. Once she reaches her goals, help her set new ones—or enjoy a maintenance program that has no further increases in the exercise but might replace some of the exercise sessions with other recreational activities.

INTENSITY

Intensity of exercise should be based on oxygen consumption. Both the oxygen delivery system and the oxygen consumption of the muscles must be challenged with an overload. This is why the recommended intensity is set at a percentage of aerobic capacity and specifically at a percentage of $\dot{V}O_2R$. Of course, unless people are exercising in a laboratory, direct knowledge of their oxygen consumption is not available. For this reason you must translate the percentage of $\dot{V}O_2R$ into a term that your client can use. There are three ways to do this:

> **Ways to Prescribe the Intensity of Aerobic Exercise**
>
> 1. Exercise prescription by heart rate
> 2. Exercise prescription by perceived exertion
> 3. Exercise prescription by workload

Regardless of the method you use, it should result in a range of intensity that falls between 50 and 85% of $\dot{V}O_2R$ (ACSM, 2006). The ACSM notes that the minimum intensity of 50% can be reduced to as low as 40% and still provide some benefit to those who start with a very low fitness level. Recent research has suggested lowering the minimum intensities from 50% to 45% $\dot{V}O_2R$ for relatively fit clients and from 40% to 30% of $\dot{V}O_2R$ for clients with a low fitness level (Swain and Franklin, 2002). The ACSM *Guidelines* acknowledge this point; thus an intensity as low as 30% $\dot{V}O_2R$ should be considered in special cases. Generally, individual clients should be prescribed an intensity range that is narrower than the overall range of 40 or 50% to 85% of $\dot{V}O_2R$. For example, you might prescribe 50 to 60% for an average client who is just beginning an exercise program, but might prescribe 70 to 80% for a more fit client.

ADDED BENEFIT OF VIGOROUS INTENSITY

When it comes to health benefits, all calories are not created equal. A review of epidemiological studies and clinical trials concluded that burning a given number of calories at a vigorous intensity, as opposed to burning the same number of calories at a moderate intensity for a longer amount of time, results in a significantly greater reduction in the risk of developing heart disease (Swain and Franklin, 2006). Reasons for the greater benefits of vigorous over moderate-intensity aerobic training include greater reduction in resting blood pressure, greater increase in aerobic capacity, and possibly better improvement in insulin sensitivity and glucose control. These improvements, and potentially others, may be related to adaptations in the autonomic nervous system. Fitness professionals routinely observe one effect of this: Highly fit clients have low resting heart rates, brought about by a change in the neural control of the heart, specifically, a reduction in sympathetic drive and increase in parasympathetic drive.

An increase in aerobic fitness may be more important in reducing coronary disease risk than merely the accumulation of a given amount of physical activity per week. Blair and colleagues found that people who increased their aerobic capacity from "unfit" (in the lowest quintile) to "fit" (any higher quintile) over a five-year period enjoyed a 52% decrease in cardiovascular mortality (Blair et al., 1995). Even those who started out with a moderate fitness level (second or third quintile) reduced their risk of mortality if they increased to a higher fitness level (fourth or fifth quintile). Each 1 MET increase in aerobic capacity was associated with a 17% reduction in mortality.

Williams performed a meta-analysis of epidemiological studies and found that people who performed the greatest amount of weekly physical activity had a 30% lower risk of developing heart disease than those who did the least amount of activity, but the risk for people with the highest aerobic capacities was 64% less than those with the lowest capacities (Williams, 2001). How could the benefit be twice as great for the highly fit people compared to the highly active people? Aren't these the same people? Not necessarily. Some people might accumulate vast amounts of caloric expenditure at a low intensity without developing a high $\dot{V}O_2$max. Therefore, available research seems to indicate that exercise prescriptions that focus on increasing $\dot{V}O_2$max may optimize cardioprotective benefits.

Figure 3.1 illustrates the effect of different training intensities on $\dot{V}O_2$max. Regardless of one's initial fitness level, training at a vigorous intensity results in greater increases in $\dot{V}O_2$max than does training at lower intensities. However, the effect is more pronounced for people who begin at a relatively high aerobic capacity. As seen in the figure, low fit people (with $\dot{V}O_2$max values below 30 ml·min^{-1}·kg^{-1}) increase their $\dot{V}O_2$max substantially when using low or moderate intensities of training, although they obtain somewhat greater increases using vigorous intensity. Relatively fit individuals (initial $\dot{V}O_2$max above 40 ml·min^{-1}·kg^{-1}) achieve no increase following low-intensity training, but receive progressively greater increases with moderate and vigorous intensities. Thus, it would

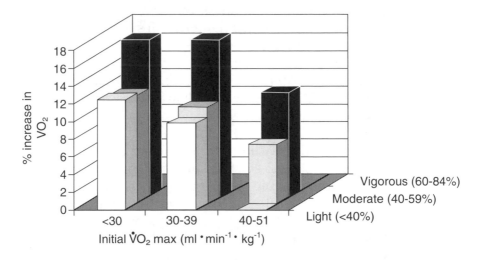

Figure 3.1 The interaction of initial fitness and exercise training intensity on the improvement in aerobic capacity. Higher intensities are more effective than lower intensities, especially for the more fit clients.

Reprinted from D.P. Swain, 2005, "Moderate or vigorous intensity exercise: Which is better for improving aerobic fitness?," *Prev. Cardiol* 8(1): 55-58, with permission of Blackwell Publishing.

be prudent to begin low fit clients with an intensity at the low end of the ACSM's recommended range. Such clients are able to reap substantial benefits at lower intensities, while minimizing the risk of orthopedic injuries, cardiovascular complications (in those with underlying disease), and burnout. However, once such clients have made significant progress, they should be encouraged to move up to higher intensities of training to obtain further increases in aerobic capacity and cardiovascular health benefits.

EXERCISE PRESCRIPTION BY HEART RATE

Heart rate varies in a linear manner with oxygen consumption during aerobic exercise. If a certain increase in oxygen demand results in a 10 bpm increase in heart rate, then twice that demand for oxygen will increase heart rate by 20 bpm. This linear response is very useful because you can measure a client's heart rate easily by palpation or by relatively inexpensive monitors. Further, because heart rate provides a good reflection of oxygen consumption, you can use it as a surrogate for oxygen consumption in writing exercise prescriptions. Remember that you are interested in the change in oxygen consumption, not the change in heart rate. A heart rate that is elevated for several minutes during a scary movie does *not* provide an aerobic training effect! Similarly, an elevated pulse during anaerobic exercise, such as weightlifting, does not indicate that an equivalent level of aerobic training stimulus is achieved. Heart rate is increased by sympathetic drive under a variety of circumstances, but it is a good indicator of oxygen consumption only if the person is engaged in aerobic exercise.

There are two popular ways to prescribe exercise intensity by heart rate: the percentage of maximal heart rate (%HRmax) method and the percentage of heart rate reserve (%HRR) method.

%HRmax Method

The %HRmax method is a simple way to calculate a target heart rate, although its exclusion of resting HR limits its usefulness to some degree. The formula for this method is simple:

Target Heart Rate by %HRmax Method:

Target HR = (intensity fraction)(HRmax)

Choose the intensity fraction to provide the appropriate intensities of $\dot{V}O_2R$. It is important to recognize that the same numerical values for %HRmax and for %$\dot{V}O_2R$ give different exercise intensities. To achieve a desired level of %$\dot{V}O_2R$, you must use a higher value for the %HRmax number. Until recently, the ACSM *Guidelines* recommended %HRmax values for exercise prescription that were too low. Fortunately, the seventh edition of the *Guidelines* revised these values upward to reflect available research (Londeree and Ames, 1976; Swain et al., 1994), and the *Guidelines* now match the values recommended in the first edition of this book and in an article by Howley (2001). Table 3.1 provides the appropriate values of %HRmax for different levels of %$\dot{V}O_2R$.

You will rarely know the true maximal heart rates of clients, but you can obtain a reasonable estimate by subtracting a person's age in years from 220 bpm. There are other formulas that may be somewhat more accurate (e.g., Tanaka et al.'s $208 - 0.7 \times$ age); however, all such formulas only provide an estimate. Approximately two-thirds of the population will have maximal heart rates that are within 10 bpm of the calculated figure (220 − age); thus, one-third will have maximal heart rates that are more than 10 bpm higher or lower than the estimate, and about 5% of normal subjects will have maximal heart rates more than 20 bpm from the estimate. For this reason, *it is much better to use a true maximal heart rate if it is*

Table 3.1   Equivalent Exercise Intensities of %$\dot{V}O_2R$, %HRR, %HRmax, and RPE for Prescribing Exercise

%$\dot{V}O_2R$	%HRR	%HRmax	RPE*
40%	40%	64%	12
50%	50%	70%	13
60%	60%	77%	14
70%	70%	84%	15
80%	80%	91%	16
85%	85%	94%	17

Cardiorespiratory exercise intensity may be prescribed as a workload (based on a desired percentage of $\dot{V}O_2R$), as a target heart rate (calculated by the %HRR method or the %HRmax method), or as a rating of perceived exertion (RPE). Percentage of HRR units provide equivalent intensities to %$\dot{V}O_2R$ units, whereas %HRmax units must be adjusted upwards to provide the same intensities.

*RPE values provide rough approximations, not "equivalent" intensities, to HR and $\dot{V}O_2$ values.

available. Although such tests are rarely performed outside a clinical environment, one can determine maximal heart rate by having a subject exercise to exhaustion in a graded exercise test.

If you do estimate maximal heart rate as 220 – age (or use other available formulas), remember that the target HR is also just an estimate. Use the target HR as a starting point, and be prepared to adjust the exercise intensity based on the client's response. After you have worked with the client, it would be appropriate to modify the target HR values based on your professional judgment.

CASE STUDY 3.2
Exercise Prescription Using %HRmax

Tawana is a 37-year-old woman who wants to enter your aerobic dance class. She has already been screened and is in the low-risk category. During the class, you will be starting with a warm-up and gradually building to a fairly vigorous routine. You tell the class participants to check their HR frequently to ensure that they are working within the target zone. Using the %HRmax method, what are Tawana's upper and lower limits of the HR range? If you use a 10-second count in your class, what number of beats should she be looking for?

Because Tawana is low risk, she can exercise anywhere within the 50 to 85% $\dot{V}O_2R$ range. She should reach or exceed the 50% level by the end of the class warm-up and should use the 85% level as an upper limit for the vigorous sections of the class. Based on table 3.1, her target HRs would be set at 70 to 94% of maximum. Her maximal HR is estimated as 220 – 37 = 183 bpm.

$$\text{Lower target HR} = (0.70)(183)$$

$$= 128 \text{ bpm}$$

$$\text{Upper target HR} = (0.94)(183)$$

$$= 172 \text{ bpm}$$

To express these targets as 10-second counts, divide the HRs in bpm by a factor of 6, yielding a range of 21 to 29 beats.

Exercise Prescription Using %HRmax

Pedro is a 24-year-old, low-risk client. He runs recreationally for three miles, four or five times per week. He finds it very difficult to maintain an even pace, especially when going up and down hills. After screening, you perform a fitness evaluation and find that his $\dot{V}O_2$max is approximately 44 ml · min^{-1} · kg^{-1}. You encourage him to purchase a heart rate monitor, using it to maintain a steady intensity rather than a steady speed. Using the %HRmax method, what HR range would you recommend for him?

Pedro has an average aerobic capacity (at the 50th percentile, based on chapter 4 of the seventh edition of ACSM's *Guidelines*). You could choose any intensity between 50 and 85% of $\dot{V}O_2$R, but it would be reasonable to narrow that down to 60 to 70% in light of his current fitness status. After he has practiced for a week with his HR monitor, you can adjust the intensity range depending on his response. According to table 3.1, the corresponding target HR range is 77 to 84% of HRmax. His estimated HRmax is $220 - 24 = 196$ bpm.

$$\text{Lower target HR} = (0.77)(196)$$

$$= 151 \text{ bpm}$$

$$\text{Upper target HR} = (0.84)(196)$$

$$= 165 \text{ bpm}$$

Because the %HRmax method of prescribing exercise intensity is so simple to use, it is very popular. Unfortunately, it is limited because it does not account for resting HR. Consider an exercise prescription for a 70-year-old woman with a resting HR of 90 bpm. If you placed her at the lowest intensity, 64% of HRmax (i.e., 40% of $\dot{V}O_2$R), the target HR would be $(0.64)(220 - 70) = 96$ bpm. The target HR is barely more than her resting HR!

Or consider an exercise prescription for two 30-year-olds, one of whom has a resting HR of 50 bpm and the other of 80 bpm. If you place both at an intensity of 70% of HRmax (i.e., 50% of $\dot{V}O_2$R), you would give both a target HR of $(0.70)(220 - 30) = 133$ bpm. However, this is an increase of 83 bpm above rest for the first client and an increase of only 53 bpm above rest for the second. Clearly, these two clients would not be exercising at the same intensity. The client with the lower resting heart rate would have a much higher relative intensity.

The heart rate reserve method avoids the problems associated with variations in resting HR.

%HRR Method

Heart rate reserve is simply the difference between resting and maximal heart rate. Because Karvonen, Kentala, and Mustala (1957) first used a percentage of this range to establish exercise intensity, this method is often called the **Karvonen method.** As chapter 2 explains, subsequent research has shown that %HRR provides intensities of exercise equivalent to the values of %$\dot{V}O_2R$. Regardless of a person's age, fitness level, or resting heart rate, the %HRR method provides accurate target heart rates relative to desired percentages of $\dot{V}O_2R$.

The formula for calculating a target HR by the %HRR method is as follows:

Target Heart Rate by %HRR Method:

Target HR = (intensity fraction)(HRmax − HRrest) + HRrest

The intensity fraction is the same numerical value as the desired percentage of $\dot{V}O_2R$. As with the %HRmax method, you can estimate maximal HR by subtracting age from 220; but always use a client's actual maximal HR if you know it. Optimally, you should measure resting HR after several (at least five) minutes of quiet rest. If the client is agitated or has just been engaged in stressful activity, the measured HR will not reflect true resting conditions. The quiet rest is best performed in a seated position, especially if the client's main form of exercise is bicycling, rowing, or some other seated activity. If the client's main form of exercise is performed in an upright posture (e.g., walking, running), it would be appropriate to have the client stand for two to three minutes after the seated rest period and then measure the HR.

Exercise Prescription Using %HRR

Jeremy is a 64-year-old, moderate-risk client. He wants to begin an exercise program to reduce his risk of heart disease. His physician has performed a stress test to evaluate his condition, and there are no indications of clinically relevant heart disease at this time. His measured maximal HR is 148 bpm, with resting HR of 86 bpm. Using the %HRR method, what would be an appropriate target HR range?

You place Jeremy at the low end of the normal intensity range, 50 to 60% of $\dot{V}O_2R$, and therefore 50 to 60% of HRR. You could estimate his maximal HR as 220 − 64 = 156 bpm, but you instead use the known value of 148 bpm. You prescribe his target HR range as follows:

$$\text{Lower target HR} = (0.50)(148 - 86) + 86$$

(Remember basic laws of algebra: First perform functions that are within parentheses; then perform multiplications or divisions; then perform additions or subtractions.)

$$= (0.50)(62) + 86$$

$$= 31 + 86$$

$$= 117 \text{ bpm}$$

$$\text{Upper target HR} = (0.60)(148 - 86) + 86$$

$$= (0.60)(62) + 86$$

$$= 37 + 86$$

$$= 123 \text{ bpm}$$

Note that if you had used the %HRmax method instead, you would have obtained the following target HRs, based on a lower limit of 70% HRmax (for 50% $\dot{V}O_2R$) and an upper limit of 77% HRmax (for 60% $\dot{V}O_2R$):

$$\text{Lower target HR} = (0.70)(148)$$

$$= 104 \text{ bpm}$$

$$\text{Upper target HR} = (0.77)(148)$$

$$= 114 \text{ bpm}$$

With a large number of clients, *average* target HRs should be similar with both %HRmax and %HRR methods. In Jeremy's case, however, the %HRmax values come out too low. The %HRR method is slightly more cumbersome mathematically, but it provides a more individually tailored prescription. Therefore it is the preferred method of prescribing HR in most settings.

EXERCISE PRESCRIPTION BY PERCEIVED EXERTION

Heart rate is an excellent measure to use for prescribing exercise intensity, but it's not for everyone. Many people can gauge the intensity of their exercise by how hard it feels. Athletes have been doing this for generations, although the use of HR monitors has recently become quite popular in certain sports. Other people may wish to use HR but may not be able to because of clinical conditions (such as cardiac transplant) or medications (such as beta-blockers) that impair the HR response to exercise. (People on beta-blockers can still use HR, provided their exercise prescription is based on HR data collected while on the medication.) Some medications (including such readily available drugs as caffeine and nicotine) may elevate rather than impair heart rate, making the heart rate prescription inaccurate.

Other conditions can also influence heart rate. For example, exercising in the heat elevates the heart rate above what would otherwise be expected, and pregnancy reduces the range of heart rates available to the exercising woman (resting HR is increased and maximal HR is reduced). Finally, some people simply find it too difficult to measure their own heart rate.

One way of prescribing exercise that relies on a person's own perception of effort is the **talk test.** If a client is still able to talk during an exercise session (i.e., can speak in complete sentences without gasping for breath), then the intensity is not excessive. Of course, this provides only an upper limit; you can describe the lower limit to a client as being "hard enough to make you aware that you are breathing harder."

The talk test effectively places most clients in an aerobic training zone, but exercise scientists have sought to quantify perceived exertion with numerical scales that provide a reasonable correlation to exercise intensity. The most popular such scale is the **rating of perceived exertion (RPE) scale** designed by Borg (1982). The scale, which ranges from 6 to 20, is intended to correspond to heart rates of 60 to 200 bpm in young adults. People of any age can use the scale, with 6 representing rest and 20 representing maximal effort. Descriptors (such as "very light" and "somewhat hard") are provided for each odd number on the scale. Clients should use the numbers or descriptors as a reflection of their *overall feeling of effort* when exercising, not just how tired their legs feel or how hard they are breathing.

The ACSM cautions that RPE scales are subjective and should be carefully compared with actual exercise intensity *on an individual basis.* Suggested RPE values are listed in table 3.1. As with any variable used to prescribe the intensity of exercise, use the RPE only as a starting point; be prepared to adjust the intensity based on the client's responses. For example, one client might report an RPE of 15 during a given exercise, yet visibly appear to be exerting very little effort. If the prescription calls for a "hard" intensity, it would be appropriate to increase the workload gradually and ask the client to reevaluate how "hard" the exercise really is.

CASE STUDY 3.5
Exercise Prescription Using RPE and %HRR

Sarah is a 42-year-old, moderate-risk client. She has a resting HR of 68 bpm. You want her to exercise at an intensity equivalent to 50 to 70% of $\dot{V}O_2R$. She finds manual measurement of HR to be difficult but says that she might purchase a HR monitor. What would be her target HR using the %HRR method, and what would be a suggested intensity range based on the Borg RPE scale?

You estimate Sarah's maximal HR as $220 - 42 = 178$ bpm. According to table 3.1, the RPE values that correspond to 50 to 70% $\dot{V}O_2R$ are 13 to 15, or "somewhat hard" to "hard." This range should correspond to the following target HRs:

$$\text{Lower target HR} = (0.50)(178 - 68) + 68$$

$$= (0.50)(110) + 68$$

$$= 55 + 68$$

$$= 123 \text{ bpm}$$

$$\text{Upper target HR} = (0.70)(178 - 68) + 68$$
$$= (0.70)(110) + 68$$
$$= 77 + 68$$
$$= 145 \text{ bpm}$$

EXERCISE PRESCRIPTION BY WORKLOAD

The third way of prescribing exercise intensity, in addition to heart rate and perceived exertion, is by workload. What would be an appropriate speed and grade on a treadmill, or resistance setting and cadence on a cycle ergometer, or wattage on a stair stepper or rowing machine? If you can tell your clients how intense the setting should be on a piece of equipment, or how fast they should be walking or jogging outdoors, then they can be at the proper exercise intensity without having to use heart rate. For clients who cannot use heart rate, exercise prescription by workload provides a more objective way to set intensity than does RPE.

Exercise scientists have performed many studies to quantify the oxygen consumption during different types of exercise. Some modes of exercise have highly predictable oxygen demands, whereas others are much more variable.

The *predictable modes of exercise* are those in which the workload is easily measured and for which the exerciser is able to maintain a steady intensity over time—walking, running, and stationary cycling. For these modes of exercise, equations have been developed that allow you to estimate the oxygen consumption with reasonable accuracy regardless of the age, sex, weight, or skill level of the exerciser (chapter 4 will discuss these equations in detail). Armed with this information, you can provide clients with appropriate workload intensities in exercise prescriptions.

The *variable forms of exercise* are those in which skill greatly affects efficiency (e.g., swimming), or in which the intensity varies throughout an exercise session. Whereas the intensity of swimming is certainly related to the speed of movement through the water, the level of skill exhibited by individual swimmers has an enormous impact on the oxygen demand, making it impossible to provide a single equation that describes the oxygen demand with accuracy.

Other examples of exercises with variable intensity are tennis, basketball, and soccer. Although people can certainly obtain a good workout through these activities, the intensity of the exercise depends on the pace of a particular game, how much effort the person chooses to use, and how much effort the opponent chooses to use. Tables have been compiled that provide general ranges of the oxygen consumption, or **MET** levels, for these activities (Ainsworth et al., 2000). Remember that *1 MET is the average oxygen consumption at rest, 3.5 ml · min^{-1} · kg^{-1}*. Thus, the MET level is the oxygen consumption expressed as multiples of resting metabolism. It is possible to use these MET tables to assign intensity in an exercise prescription. However, because people choose to use quite variable levels of effort, the potential ranges of intensity in such activities are much greater than even the tables indicate—making prescription by this method of limited value. You can make accurate intensity prescriptions only for the highly predictable modes of aerobic exercise. Chapter 4 will introduce the mathematical equations used to quantify the workload in such cases.

REFERENCES

ACSM. 2006. *ACSM's Guidelines for Exercise Testing and Prescription*, 7th ed., 133-173. Philadelphia: Lippincott Williams & Wilkins.

Ainsworth, B.E., W.L. Haskell, M.C. Whitt, M.L. Irwin, A.M. Swartz, S.J. Strath, W.L. O'Brien, D.R. Bassett, K.H. Schmitz, P.O. Emplaincourt, D.R. Jacobs, and A.S. Leon. 2000. Compendium of physical activities: An update of activity codes and MET intensities. *Medicine and Science in Sports and Exercise* 32 (9 Suppl.): S498-504.

Blair, S.N., H.W. Kohl, C.E. Barlow, R.S. Paffenbarger, L.W. Gibbons, and C.A. Macera. 1995. Changes in physical fitness and all-cause mortality. *Journal of the American Medical Association* 273: 1093-1098.

Borg, G. 1982. Psychophysical bases of perceived exertion. *Medicine and Science in Sports and Exercise* 14: 377-381.

Howley, E.T. 2001. Type of activity: Resistance, aerobic, anaerobic and leisure time versus occupational physical activity. *Medicine and Science in Sports and Exercise* 33 (6 Suppl.): 364-369.

Karvonen, M.J., E. Kentala, and O. Mustala. 1957. The effects of training on heart rate: A longitudinal study. *Annales Medicinae Experimentalis et Biologiae Fenniae* 35: 307-315.

Londeree, B.R., and S.A. Ames. 1976. Trend analysis of the %$\dot{V}O_2$max-HR regression. *Medicine and Science in Sports and Exercise* 8: 122-125.

Swain, D.P. 2005. Moderate or vigorous intensity exercise: Which is better for improving aerobic fitness? *Preventive Cardiology* 8: 55-58.

Swain, D.P., K.S. Abernathy, C.S. Smith, S.J. Lee, and S.A. Bunn. 1994. Target heart rates for the development of cardiorespiratory fitness. *Medicine and Science in Sports and Exercise* 26: 112-116.

Swain, D.P., and B.A. Franklin. 2002. $\dot{V}O_2$ Reserve and the minimal intensity for improving cardiorespiratory fitness. *Medicine and Science in Sports and Exercise* 34: 152-157.

Swain, D.P., and B.A. Franklin. 2006. Comparative cardioprotective benefits of vigorous vs. moderate intensity aerobic exercise. *American Journal of Cardiology* 97 (1): 141-147.

Tanaka, H., K.D. Monahan, and D. R. Seals. 2001. Age-predicted maximal heart rate revisited. *Journal of the American College of Cardiology* 37:153-156.

Williams, P.T. 2001. Physical fitness and activity as separate heart disease risk factors: A meta-analysis. *Medicine and Science in Sports and Exercise* 33: 754-761.

4

Using the ACSM
Metabolic Equations

The ACSM has developed equations for estimating oxygen consumption during walking, running, stationary cycling, and stepping (ACSM, 2006). The equations are reasonably accurate for a wide range of people, because age, sex, and skill do not strongly affect the energy demands of these modes of exercise. Body size does affect the energy demands, but this is accounted for in the equations.

The ACSM equations are fairly accurate, but they are only estimates. Therefore, workload prescriptions or weight loss calculations based on these equations are estimates as well. As with prescriptions that use heart rate or perceived exertion to establish intensity, always observe a client's responses to the prescribed workload and be prepared to make adjustments.

The ACSM's equations are modified every few years, as new research warrants. When the ACSM's *Guidelines* were developed for the sixth edition, one of the authors of this book (Swain) made several modifications to the equations: A term for unloaded cycling (the oxygen cost of moving the legs themselves) was added to the leg cycling equation, a term for resting metabolism was added to the stepping equation, and all equations were formatted to yield answers for oxygen consumption in the units ml $\cdot$ min^{-1} $\cdot$ kg^{-1} (Swain, 2000). For the seventh edition of the *Guidelines*, there was one formatting change: The workload term in the leg and arm cycling equations was presented in kg $\cdot$ m $\cdot$ min^{-1} rather than watts. This book uses the equations that appear in the ACSM's seventh edition; they are summarized on the next page.

The ACSM's Metabolic Equations

Walking
$\dot{V}O_2 = 3.5 + 0.1(\text{speed}) + 1.8(\text{speed})(\text{fractional grade})$

Running
$\dot{V}O_2 = 3.5 + 0.2(\text{speed}) + 0.9(\text{speed})(\text{fractional grade})$

Leg cycling
$\dot{V}O_2 = 7 + 1.8(\text{work rate})/(\text{body mass})$

Arm cycling
$\dot{V}O_2 = 3.5 + 3(\text{work rate})/(\text{body mass})$

Stepping
$\dot{V}O_2 = 3.5 + 0.2(\text{stepping rate}) + 2.4(\text{stepping rate})(\text{step height})$

Where:
$\dot{V}O_2$ is in ml $\cdot$ min^{-1} $\cdot$ kg^{-1}
Speed is in m $\cdot$ min^{-1}
Work rate is in kg $\cdot$ m $\cdot$ min^{-1}
Body mass is in kg
Stepping rate is in steps per min
Step height is in m

Adapted, by permission, from American College of Sports Medicine (ACSM), 2006, *ACSM's guidelines for exercise testing and prescription*, 7th ed. (Philadelphia, PA: Lippincott Williams & Wilkins), 289.

FUNCTIONS OF THE METABOLIC EQUATIONS

You can use the metabolic equations for two purposes. *First, use them to calculate the oxygen consumption, and thus the energy expenditure, of a specific exercise.* This is valuable when you want to determine how many calories a client is burning during an exercise session and how much weight loss can be anticipated. *Second, you can use the equations to calculate the target workload in an exercise prescription.* When heart rate or RPE may not be preferred, you can tell your client the intensity of exercise as a specific workload on a piece of exercise equipment or as a walking or running speed outdoors.

The metabolic equations yield oxygen consumption in gross terms. That is, they provide a person's *total* oxygen consumption, including both the $\dot{V}O_2$ needed for resting metabolism and the additional $\dot{V}O_2$ needed for the exercise itself. To determine the *net* $\dot{V}O_2$, for example, when determining the number of calories that an exercise session expends above rest, simply subtract 3.5 ml · min^{-1} · kg^{-1} from the gross value.

$$\text{Gross } \dot{V}O_2 = \text{resting } \dot{V}O_2 + \text{exercise } \dot{V}O_2$$

$$\text{Gross } \dot{V}O_2 = 3.5 \text{ ml} \cdot min^{-1} \cdot kg^{-1} + \text{net } \dot{V}O_2$$

$$\text{Net } \dot{V}O_2 = \text{gross } \dot{V}O_2 - 3.5 \text{ ml} \cdot min^{-1} \cdot kg^{-1}$$

CONVERSION OF UNITS

Depending on the situation, some of the terms used in the ACSM metabolic equations may not be in appropriate units. For example, rather than expressing oxygen consumption in ml · min^{-1} · kg^{-1}, one might need to express it in L · min^{-1}, or in METs, or even in kcal · min^{-1} of energy expenditure. Likewise, you may need to alter the units for workload in the various equations. For example, speed is indicated in m · min^{-1}, but you might prefer mph or kph. And cycling workload is in kg · m · min^{-1} (which is not technically power); you may prefer a measurement using watts. Table 4.1 provides the factors for converting between these various units.

Here is the simplest approach to using the equations:

1. Convert any raw data into the units as they appear in the equations.

2. Solve the equation using basic algebra.

3. If necessary, convert the answer into desired units.

This approach is followed in case studies later in this chapter.

WALKING

The energy cost of walking increases in direct proportion with speed over the normal range of walking speeds. When a person tries to walk *extremely* fast, the energy cost increases exponentially. Thus, the walking equation should be used only for normal

Table 4.1   Conversion Factors for Metabolic Equations

$\dfrac{(\dot{V}O_2 \text{ in } L \cdot min^{-1}) \times 1{,}000}{\text{body mass}} = \dot{V}O_2 \text{ in } ml \cdot min^{-1} \cdot kg^{-1}$	$\dfrac{(\dot{V}O_2 \text{ in } ml \cdot min^{-1} \cdot kg^{-1})(\text{body mass})}{1{,}000} = \dot{V}O_2 \text{ in } L \cdot min^{-1}$
$(\dot{V}O_2 \text{ in METs}) \times 3.5 = \dot{V}O_2 \text{ in } ml \cdot min^{-1} \cdot kg^{-1}$	$\dfrac{(\dot{V}O_2 \text{ in } ml \cdot min^{-1} \cdot kg^{-1})}{3.5} = \dot{V}O_2 \text{ in METs}$
$(\dot{V}O_2 \text{ in } L \cdot min^{-1}) \times 5 = \text{energy exp. in } kcal \cdot min^{-1}$	$\dfrac{\text{energy exp. in } kcal \cdot min^{-1}}{5} = \dot{V}O_2 \text{ in } L \cdot min^{-1}$
$(\text{speed in mph}) \times 26.8 = \text{speed in } m \cdot min^{-1}$	$\dfrac{\text{speed in } m \cdot min^{-1}}{26.8} = \text{speed in mph}$
$\dfrac{\text{speed in kph}}{0.06} = \text{speed in } m \cdot min^{-1}$	$(\text{speed in } m \cdot min^{-1}) \times 0.06 = \text{speed in kph}$
$\dfrac{\text{work rate in } kg \cdot m \cdot min^{-1}}{6} = \text{power in W}$	$(\text{power in W}) \times 6 = \text{work rate in } kg \cdot m \cdot min^{-1}$

(Note: $kg \cdot m \cdot min^{-1}$ is not technically a unit of power; also, conversion with the acceleration of gravity yields a correction factor of 6.12; however, the ACSM uses 6 as a reasonable approximation for exercise prescriptions.)

$(\text{weight in lb}) \times 2.2 = \text{mass in kg}$	$\dfrac{\text{mass in kg}}{2.2} = \text{weight in lb}$

(Note: Pounds are not a unit of mass but can be converted with the factor 2.2 when the mass in question is subject to earth's gravity; for greater precision, a factor of 2.2046 can be used.)

$(\text{height in inches}) \times 0.0254 = \text{height in m}$	$\dfrac{\text{height in m}}{0.0254} = \text{height in inches}$

walking speeds, not race walking. The equation is accurate for treadmill or overground walking. When walking on flat ground (i.e., the grade is zero), the last term in the equation drops out. The equation cannot be used for walking downhill. The energy cost of downhill walking varies in a U-shaped curve with grade. Walking down slight downhill slopes requires less energy than level walking, because of the assistance of gravity. The minimum cost is about half that of level walking and occurs at approximately a 10% decline. As the slope becomes steeper, the energy cost increases; it becomes greater than the cost of level walking for declines greater than 20% (Minetti et al., 2002). The increased energy cost with steeper descents is likely due to greater effort in braking.

Walking—Solve for the $\dot{V}O_2$

George is a 51-year-old, moderate-risk client who weighs 163 lb. Because of his high-stress job, he has recently started an exercise program in the company wellness facility. He has selected his treadmill workload at a comfortable level, which is walking at 3 mph up a 6% grade. What is his estimated gross oxygen consumption in ml·min^{-1}·kg^{-1}, and what is the net number of calories he is burning each minute?

Convert any terms into the units requested by the equations (speed in mph to m·min^{-1}, and weight in lb to mass in kg). Select the appropriate conversion factors from table 4.1.

$$3 \text{ mph} \times 26.8 = 80.4 \text{ m·min}^{-1}$$

$$163 \text{ lb} / 2.2 = 74.1 \text{ kg}$$

Second, select the walking equation from the list on page 50, enter all of the known variables, and solve for the unknown $\dot{V}O_2$. Remember to enter the grade as a fraction (0.06), not in percent units.

$$\dot{V}O_2 = 3.5 + 0.1(\text{speed}) + 1.8(\text{speed})(\text{fractional grade})$$

$$= 3.5 + 0.1(80.4) + 1.8(80.4)(0.06)$$

(In solving algebraic equations, always perform multiplications or divisions before additions or subtractions.)

$$= 3.5 + 8.04 + 8.6832$$

$$= 20.2 \text{ ml·min}^{-1}\text{·kg}^{-1}$$

George is exercising with a gross $\dot{V}O_2$ of a little more than 20 ml·min^{-1}·kg^{-1}. To determine his net caloric expenditure, first subtract resting oxygen consumption from the gross value:

$$\text{Net } \dot{V}O_2 = 20.2 - 3.5 = 16.7 \text{ ml·min}^{-1}\text{·kg}^{-1}$$

If you had wanted net $\dot{V}O_2$ at the outset, you could simply have dropped the 3.5 from the walking equation when you first solved the problem.

Third, convert this oxygen consumption to a caloric expenditure. As seen in table 4.1, there is no direct conversion between

(continued)

ml · min^{-1} · kg^{-1} and kcal · min^{-1}. But there is an intermediate term, L · min^{-1}, that can serve as a bridge between the two.

$$\frac{(16.7 \text{ ml} \cdot \text{min}^{-1} \cdot \text{kg}^{-1}) \ (74.1 \text{ kg})}{1,000} = 1.237 \text{ L} \cdot \text{min}^{-1}$$

$$(1.237 \text{ L} \cdot \text{min}^{-1}) \times 5 = 6.2 \text{ kcal} \cdot \text{min}^{-1}$$

During his treadmill walking, George is burning approximately 6.2 kcal per minute above his resting energy expenditure.

CASE STUDY 4.2
Walking—Solve for the Workload

Jonathan is a 34-year-old heart transplant patient whose heart rate varies very little from rest to exercise. He has a $\dot{V}O_2$max of 32 ml · min^{-1} · kg^{-1}. His physician has referred him to your facility for exercise training and wants him to begin at an intensity between 40 and 60% of $\dot{V}O_2$R. You have found that Jonathan walks comfortably at 2.5 mph. What treadmill grades would allow him to exercise at the desired intensity range?

First, put all terms into the desired units. Convert the walking speed into m · min^{-1}. Also, determine what values for $\dot{V}O_2$ will be entered into the walking equation using the $\dot{V}O_2$R formula from chapter 2.

$$2.5 \text{ mph} \times 26.8 = 67 \text{ m} \cdot \text{min}^{-1}$$

$$\text{Target } \dot{V}O_2 = (\text{intensity fraction})(\dot{V}O_2\text{max} - 3.5) + 3.5$$

$$\text{Lower target } \dot{V}O_2 = (0.40)(32 - 3.5) + 3.5$$

$$= (0.40)(28.5) + 3.5$$

$$= 11.4 + 3.5$$

$$= 14.9 \text{ ml} \cdot \text{min}^{-1} \cdot \text{kg}^{-1}$$

$$\text{Upper target } \dot{V}O_2 = (0.60)(32 - 3.5) + 3.5$$

$$= (0.60)(28.5) + 3.5$$

$$= 17.1 + 3.5$$

$$= 20.6 \text{ ml} \cdot \text{min}^{-1} \cdot \text{kg}^{-1}$$

Second, select the walking equation from page 50, enter the known values, and solve for the unknown grade. Do this twice, once for the lower target and once for the upper target. Doing the lower target first:

$$\dot{V}O_2 = 3.5 + 0.1(\text{speed}) + 1.8(\text{speed})(\text{fractional grade})$$

$$14.9 = 3.5 + 0.1(67) + 1.8(67)(\text{fractional grade})$$

To solve this equation, first simplify all the terms, doing multiplications first.

$$14.9 = 3.5 + 6.7 + 120.6(\text{fractional grade})$$

Continue to simplify, by doing the available addition on the right side of the equation.

$$14.9 = 10.2 + 120.6(\text{fractional grade})$$

The terms within the equation cannot be simplified any further. Now isolate the unknown, fractional grade, on its side of the equation. To do this, remove loosely attached terms first—that is, those that are being added or subtracted with the unknown. Then remove more tightly attached terms—those that are being multiplied or divided with the unknown.

$$14.9 - 10.2 = 120.6(\text{fractional grade})$$

$$4.7 = 120.6(\text{fractional grade})$$

Now, remove the 120.6 from the right side of the equation by dividing both sides with that value.

$$4.7 / 120.6 = \text{fractional grade}$$

$$0.039 = \text{fractional grade}$$

$$\text{or, } 3.9\% \text{ grade}$$

The lower target $\dot{V}O_2$ would be achieved by walking at 2.5 mph (4 kph) up a treadmill set at approximately 4%. Now, solve for the upper target.

$$20.6 = 3.5 + 0.1(67) + 1.8(67)(\text{fractional grade})$$

(The right side of the equation was simplified earlier, so just copy that from there.)

(continued)

Case Study 4.2   *(continued)*

20.6 = 10.2 + 120.6(fractional grade)

(Now, solve for the unknown.)

20.6 – 10.2 = 120.6(fractional grade)

10.4 = 120.6(fractional grade)

10.4 / 120.6 = fractional grade

0.086 = fractional grade

or, 8.6% grade

Jonathan can achieve the proper intensity in his exercise prescription by walking at 2.5 mph on a treadmill at approximately a 4 to 9% grade.

RUNNING

Running on a level surface requires twice the effort as walking, because of the extra work of literally jumping from one foot to the other. To account for this extra work, the horizontal component of the running equation (0.2 ml of O_2 for each m traveled) is twice that for walking. In contrast, the vertical component for running up a grade is only half that for walking (0.9 vs. 1.8 ml of O_2 for each kg · m of work).

The difference in the vertical components for walking and running has been a source of confusion. Shouldn't the work of lifting a given amount of body mass a certain distance up a grade be the same, regardless of how one does it? This disparity has often been erroneously explained as an anomaly associated with treadmills: A walker is in constant contact with the treadmill belt, whereas a runner is airborne between strides, with the treadmill belt sliding beneath. The explanation given was that this loss of contact with the moving belt must mean that the runner wasn't actually climbing as much as a walker on a treadmill or as much as either a walker or a runner on an outdoor hill. Well, this explanation was wrong. A research study, which had been overlooked for several years (Bassett et al., 1985), compared running up a hill and running up a treadmill—and found that they have the same oxygen cost, which is less than the vertical component for walking.

So why is the vertical component for running less than it is for walking? During level running, the runner jumps into the air to land on the opposite foot. Apparently, some of the vertical movement that normally occurs during level running is used for the ascent of a grade. The single equation for running that appears on page 50 can be used for running on a treadmill or for running outdoors. However, it cannot be used for downhill running. As described for downhill walking, downhill running is easier on slight declines and harder on steep declines (Minetti et al., 2002).

CASE STUDY 4.3
Running—Solve for the V̇O₂

Alexandra is a 26-year-old, low-risk client who weighs 118 lb. She is running on a treadmill at 7 mph up a 3% grade. What is her gross oxygen consumption in METs, and what is her net caloric expenditure?

First, convert terms into the units used by the metabolic equations.

$$7 \text{ mph} \times 26.8 = 187.6 \text{ m} \cdot \text{min}^{-1}$$

$$118 \text{ lb} / 2.2 = 53.6 \text{ kg}$$

Second, select the running equation from page 50, enter the known variables, and solve for the unknown V̇O₂.

$$\dot{V}O_2 = 3.5 + 0.2(\text{speed}) + 0.9(\text{speed})(\text{fractional grade})$$

$$= 3.5 + 0.2(187.6) + 0.9(187.6)(0.03)$$

$$= 3.5 + 37.52 + 5.0652$$

$$= 46.1 \text{ ml} \cdot \text{min}^{-1} \cdot \text{kg}^{-1}$$

Third, convert the answer into the requested terms (i.e., the gross number of METs and the net kcal · min⁻¹). To convert from ml · min⁻¹ · kg⁻¹ to METs, use the conversion factor in table 4.1.

$$(46.1 \text{ ml} \cdot \text{min}^{-1} \cdot \text{kg}^{-1}) / 3.5 = 13.2 \text{ METs}$$

(continued)

Case Study 4.3   *(continued)*

Alexandra is exercising at 13.2 METs, a little more than 13 times resting metabolism. To convert from ml · min^{-1} · kg^{-1} to kcal · min^{-1}, use the intermediate term of L · min^{-1}. But first, subtract 3.5 ml · min^{-1} · kg^{-1}, because the caloric expenditure was requested as a net value.

$$\text{Net } \dot{V}O_2 = 46.1 - 3.5 = 42.6 \text{ ml · min}^{-1} \cdot \text{kg}^{-1}$$

Converting to L · min^{-1}:

$$\frac{(42.6 \text{ ml · min}^{-1} \cdot \text{kg}^{-1})(53.6 \text{ kg})}{1,000} = 2.283 \text{ L · min}^{-1}$$

And now, converting to kcal · min^{-1}:

$$(2.283 \text{ L · min}^{-1}) \times 5 = 11.4 \text{ kcal · min}^{-1}$$

Alexandra is burning approximately 11.4 kcal · min^{-1} above resting energy expenditure when she runs on a treadmill at 7 mph up a 3% grade.

CASE STUDY 4.4
Running—Solve for the Workload

Jeannie is a 57-year-old competitive runner. She is technically in the moderate-risk category because of her age, but she is very fit and healthy, running 50 to 60 miles per week. Most of her running is on flat ground, and she competes in distance races at a pace of about 6:30 per mile. She would like to know what sort of pace she should try to maintain on a long hill in an upcoming race. The hill has an average grade of 8%. She has a measured $\dot{V}O_2$max of 62 ml · min^{-1} · kg^{-1}. Assuming that she can run at 75 to 85% of $\dot{V}O_2$R for extended periods of time, what speed (and pace per mile) should she anticipate for this hill?

First, you must calculate the value for $\dot{V}O_2$ from the desired percentage of $\dot{V}O_2$R. Do this twice, once for the lower target and once for the upper target.

$$\text{Lower target } \dot{V}O_2 = 0.75(62 - 3.5) + 3.5$$
$$= 0.75(58.5) + 3.5$$
$$= 43.9 + 3.5$$
$$= 47.4 \text{ ml} \cdot \text{min}^{-1} \cdot \text{kg}^{-1}$$

$$\text{Upper target } \dot{V}O_2 = 0.85(62 - 3.5) + 3.5$$
$$= 0.85(58.5) + 3.5$$
$$= 49.7 + 3.5$$
$$= 53.2 \text{ ml} \cdot \text{min}^{-1} \cdot \text{kg}^{-1}$$

Second, select the running equation from page 50, enter the known values, and solve for the unknown speed. First, do this for the lower target:

$$\dot{V}O_2 = 3.5 + 0.2(\text{speed}) + 0.9(\text{speed})(\text{fractional grade})$$
$$47.4 = 3.5 + 0.2(\text{speed}) + 0.9(\text{speed})(0.08)$$
$$47.4 = 3.5 + 0.2(\text{speed}) + 0.072(\text{speed})$$
$$47.4 = 3.5 + (0.2 + 0.072)(\text{speed})$$
$$47.4 = 3.5 + 0.272(\text{speed})$$
$$47.4 - 3.5 = 0.272(\text{speed})$$
$$43.9 = 0.272(\text{speed})$$
$$43.9 / 0.272 = \text{speed}$$
$$161.4 \text{ m} \cdot \text{min}^{-1} = \text{speed}$$

Now, the upper target:

$$53.2 = 3.5 + 0.2(\text{speed}) + 0.9(\text{speed})(0.08)$$
$$53.2 = 3.5 + 0.272(\text{speed})$$
$$53.2 - 3.5 = 0.272(\text{speed})$$
$$49.7 = 0.272(\text{speed})$$
$$49.7 / 0.272 = \text{speed}$$
$$182.7 \text{ m} \cdot \text{min}^{-1} = \text{speed}$$

(continued)

Case Study 4.4   *(continued)*

Third, convert the answer into the desired units—in this case, miles per hour and minutes per mile. To convert from m · min^{-1} to mph, use the conversion factor in table 4.1.

Lower target speed:

$$(161.4 \text{ m} \cdot \text{min}^{-1}) / 26.8 = 6.0 \text{ mph}$$

Upper target speed:

$$(182.7 \text{ m} \cdot \text{min}^{-1}) / 26.8 = 6.8 \text{ mph}$$

To convert miles per hour to a pace in minutes per mile, simply divide the miles per hour into 60, and then convert the fractional number of minutes into seconds.

Lower target pace:

$$(60 \text{ min per hr}) / (6.0 \text{ miles per hr}) = 10 \text{ min per mile}$$

Upper target pace:

$$60 / 6.8 = 8.82 \text{ min per mile}$$

$$= 8 \text{ min} + 0.82 \times 60 \text{ s per mile}$$

$$= 8 \text{ min and } 49 \text{ s per mile}$$

Jeannie can expect to run up the 8% hill at a pace between 8:49 and 10:00, as opposed to her 6:30 pace on flat ground.

LEG CYCLING

As mentioned earlier, the leg cycling equation includes a term for unloaded cycling. Pedaling a bike with no resistance is noticeably more work than sitting still. The mass of the legs is substantial, and moving them in a circle at 50 to 60 rpm requires about 1 additional MET (i.e., 3.5 ml · min^{-1} · kg^{-1}) of oxygen consumption (Lang et al., 1992; Latin and Berg, 1994; Londeree et al., 1997). The metabolic equation on page 50 has already added the resting and unloaded cycling terms together, yielding a single term of 7 ml · min^{-1} · kg^{-1}. The factor for loaded cycling is 1.8 ml of oxygen for each kg · m of work, which is the same as the value for vertical work in the walking and stepping equations.

Obviously, if people spin their legs faster than 60 rpm, the oxygen cost of unloaded cycling will be higher. However, research has shown that the factor for loaded cycling decreases in a compensating way as cadence increases (Londeree et al., 1997), making the single equation reasonably accurate for cadences up to at least 90 rpm.

Laboratory cycle ergometers generally do not have a power readout but simply indicate the resistance setting (in kg) and the cadence. You can determine the workload (also termed "work rate") for ergometers from the following equation:

Cycle ergometry work rate equation:

Work rate = (resistance setting)(flywheel distance per revolution)(rpm)

In this formula, the work rate is in the units $kg \cdot m \cdot min^{-1}$, and the distance that the flywheel travels for one pedal revolution is in meters. This value is 6 m for the Monark leg ergometers and 3 m for BodyGuard and Tunturi ergometers. Many exercise cycles have a power readout in watts. *One watt is equivalent to approximately $6 \ kg \cdot m \cdot min^{-1}$.*

CASE STUDY 4.5
Leg Cycling—Solve for the $\dot{V}O_2$

Marvin is a 37-year-old, 173 lb, moderate-risk client who is exercising to lose weight. He cycles on a Monark ergometer at 50 rpm with a resistance setting of 3 kg. How many minutes would he need to cycle to burn off the calories in one pound of fat?

First, put all of the relevant terms into the units called for by the leg cycling equation. You need to convert the body weight to a body mass and determine the work rate in $kg \cdot m \cdot min^{-1}$.

173 lb / 2.2 = 78.6 kg

Work rate = (resistance setting)(flywheel distance per rev)(rpm)

= (3 kg)(6 m)(50 rpm)

= 900 kg $\cdot$ m $\cdot$ min^{-1}

Second, select the leg cycling equation from page 50, enter the known values, and solve for the unknown $\dot{V}O_2$:

(continued)

Case Study 4.5   *(continued)*

$$\dot{V}O_2 = 7 + 1.8\text{(work rate)} / \text{(body mass)}$$

$$= 7 + 1.8(900) / 78.6$$

$$= 7 + 1620 / 78.6$$

$$= 7 + 20.6$$

$$= 27.6 \text{ ml} \cdot \text{min}^{-1} \cdot \text{kg}^{-1}$$

Third, because the question concerns weight loss, express the $\dot{V}O_2$ as a net value. Then convert it to $L \cdot \text{min}^{-1}$ and finally to kcal $\cdot$ min^{-1}:

$$\text{Net } \dot{V}O_2 = 27.6 - 3.5 = 24.1 \text{ ml} \cdot \text{min}^{-1} \cdot \text{kg}^{-1}$$

$$\frac{(24.1 \text{ ml} \cdot \text{min}^{-1} \cdot \text{kg}^{-1})(78.6 \text{ kg})}{1,000} = 1.894 \text{ L} \cdot \text{min}^{-1}$$

$$(1.894 \text{ L} \cdot \text{min}^{-1}) \times 5 = 9.47 \text{ kcal} \cdot \text{min}^{-1}$$

One pound of fat contains approximately 3,500 kcal of stored energy, so Marvin would need to accumulate 3,500 / 9.47 = 370 minutes of this exercise (a little over 6 hr) to lose one pound (assuming all calories burned by the exercise are in excess of dietary intake).

CASE STUDY 4.6
Leg Cycling—Solve for the Workload

Abigail is a 42-year-old, moderate-risk client who weighs 147 lb. You have estimated her $\dot{V}O_2$max as 29 ml $\cdot$ min^{-1} $\cdot$ kg^{-1} and would like her to exercise at 60 to 70% of $\dot{V}O_2$R. She has purchased a stationary bike that has a power readout in watts. What would be an appropriate target intensity range for her on this bike?

First, convert terms. In this case, convert her body weight into a body mass and determine her lower and upper target $\dot{V}O_2$s using the $\dot{V}O_2$R formula:

$$147 \text{ lb} / 2.2 = 66.8 \text{ kg}$$

$$\text{Target } \dot{V}O_2 = (\text{intensity fraction})(\dot{V}O_2\text{max} - 3.5) + 3.5$$

$$\text{Lower target } \dot{V}O_2 = (0.60)(29 - 3.5) + 3.5$$

$$= (0.60)(25.5) + 3.5$$

$$= 15.3 + 3.5$$

$$= 18.8 \text{ ml} \cdot \text{min}^{-1} \cdot \text{kg}^{-1}$$

$$\text{Upper target } \dot{V}O_2 = (0.70)(29 - 3.5) + 3.5$$

$$= (0.70)(25.5) + 3.5$$

$$= 17.85 + 3.5$$

$$= 21.4 \text{ ml} \cdot \text{min}^{-1} \cdot \text{kg}^{-1}$$

Second, select the leg cycling equation from page 50, enter the known values, and solve for the unknown workload:
Lower target workload:

$$\dot{V}O_2 = 7 + 1.8(\text{work rate}) / (\text{body mass})$$

$$18.8 = 7 + 1.8(\text{work rate}) / 66.8$$

(There are three numbers associated with the unknown. To isolate it, remove the most loosely attached term first, the one that is being added.)

$$18.8 - 7 = 1.8(\text{work rate}) / 66.8$$

$$11.8 = 1.8(\text{work rate}) / 66.8$$

(Now, remove the other two terms to isolate the unknown. It doesn't matter which is done first. In this example, first multiply both sides by the body mass, and then divide both sides by the work rate coefficient.)

$$11.8 \times 66.8 = 1.8(\text{work rate})$$

$$788.24 = 1.8(\text{work rate})$$

$$788.24 / 1.8 = \text{work rate}$$

$$437.9 \text{ kg} \cdot \text{m} \cdot \text{min}^{-1} = \text{work rate}$$

(continued)

Case Study 4.6   *(continued)*

Upper target workload:

$$21.4 = 7 + 1.8(\text{work rate}) / 66.8$$

$$21.4 - 7 = 1.8(\text{work rate}) / 66.8$$

$$14.4 = 1.8(\text{work rate}) / 66.8$$

$$14.4 \times 66.8 = 1.8(\text{work rate})$$

$$961.92 = 1.8(\text{work rate})$$

$$961.92 / 1.8 = \text{work rate}$$

$$534.4 \text{ kg} \cdot \text{m} \cdot \text{min}^{-1} = \text{work rate}$$

Third, convert the answer into the desired units. To convert kg · m · min^{-1} to W, divide the former by 6.

Lower target workload:

$$(437.9 \text{ kg} \cdot \text{m} \cdot \text{min}^{-1}) / 6 = 73 \text{ W}$$

Upper target workload:

$$(534.4 \text{ kg} \cdot \text{m} \cdot \text{min}^{-1}) / 6 = 89 \text{ W}$$

Abigail can exercise in her target intensity range by cycling at approximately 73 to 89 W.

ARM CYCLING

The ACSM's arm cycling metabolic equation does not include a term for unloaded cycling. At this time, available research does not suggest that such a term is needed (Franklin, 1985), possibly because of the small mass of the arms as compared to the legs. An important consideration in arm cycling is that it requires significantly more oxygen consumption than leg cycling to perform the same workload, as indicated by the factor of 3 ml of oxygen per kg · m, instead of 1.8 for the legs. It is believed that the higher factor for the arms is due to less efficiency in performing a given amount of work with a smaller muscle mass.

When using a laboratory arm ergometer, always check the flywheel distance before calculating the workload. Monark arm ergometers have a flywheel distance of 2.4 m.

Arm Cycling—Solve for the $\dot{V}O_2$

Akiko is a 61-year-old, 127 lb coronary bypass patient. During her phase II rehabilitation, she is introduced to the use of a Monark arm ergometer. She is asked to select a comfortable resistance level while cranking at 50 rpm, keeping her HR within a range prescribed by her physician. After warming up, she uses a resistance of 1 kg. What is her estimated oxygen consumption during this exercise?

First, convert terms to appropriate units. In this case, convert her body weight to body mass and determine her workload on the arm ergometer in kg·m·min^{-1}.

$$127 \text{ lb} / 2.2 = 57.7 \text{ kg}$$

Work rate = (resistance setting)(flywheel distance per rev)(rpm)

$$= (1 \text{ kg})(2.4 \text{ m})(50 \text{ rpm})$$

$$= 120 \text{ kg·m·min}^{-1}$$

Second, select the arm cycling equation from page 50, enter the known values, and solve for the unknown $\dot{V}O_2$:

$$\dot{V}O_2 = 3.5 + 3(\text{work rate}) / (\text{body mass})$$

$$= 3.5 + 3(120) / 57.7$$

$$= 3.5 + 360 / 57.7$$

$$= 3.5 + 6.2$$

$$= 9.7 \text{ ml·min}^{-1}\text{·kg}^{-1}$$

Akiko is exercising with a gross $\dot{V}O_2$ of approximately 9.7 ml·min^{-1}·kg^{-1} on the arm ergometer.

Arm Cycling—Solve for the Workload

Fred is an 18-year-old, 152 lb male who had a spinal injury in a car accident six months ago and is now paraplegic. You are prescribing an exercise program for him on a Monark arm ergometer. His $\dot{V}O_2$max (recently measured on an arm ergometer) is 28.5 ml·min^{-1}·kg^{-1}, and you want him to begin his exercise program at 50% of

(continued)

Case Study 4.8   *(continued)*

$\dot{V}O_2R$. What is the appropriate workload on the arm ergometer? You have found that he prefers to crank on the ergometer at a cadence of 70 rpm. What resistance setting should he use to achieve the desired workload?

First, convert his body weight into body mass and determine his target $\dot{V}O_2$ using the $\dot{V}O_2R$ formula:

$$152 \text{ lb}/2.2 = 69.1 \text{ kg}$$

$$\text{Target } \dot{V}O_2 = (\text{intensity fraction})(\dot{V}O_2\text{max} - 3.5) + 3.5$$

$$= (0.50)(28.5 - 3.5) + 3.5$$

$$= (0.50)(25) + 3.5$$

$$= 12.5 + 3.5$$

$$= 16.0 \text{ ml} \cdot \text{min}^{-1} \cdot \text{kg}^{-1}$$

Second, select the arm cycling equation from page 50, enter the known values, and solve for the unknown workload:

$$\dot{V}O_2 = 3.5 + 3(\text{work rate}) / (\text{body mass})$$

$$16.0 = 3.5 + 3(\text{work rate}) / 69.1$$

$$16.0 - 3.5 = 3(\text{work rate}) / 69.1$$

$$12.5 = 3(\text{work rate}) / 69.1$$

$$12.5 \times 69.1 = 3(\text{work rate})$$

$$863.75 = 3(\text{work rate})$$

$$863.75 / 3 = \text{work rate}$$

$$288 \text{ kg} \cdot \text{m} \cdot \text{min}^{-1} = \text{work rate}$$

Fred's workload should be a little less than 290 kg · m · min⁻¹. If he cranks the arm ergometer at 70 rpm, his resistance setting would be as follows:

$$\text{Work rate} = (\text{resistance setting})(\text{flywheel distance per rev})(\text{rpm})$$

$$288 = (\text{resistance setting})(2.4)(70)$$

$$288 = (\text{resistance setting})(168)$$

$$288 / 168 = \text{resistance setting}$$

$$1.7 \text{ kg} = \text{resistance setting}$$

STEPPING

The ACSM's stepping equation was modified for the sixth edition of the *Guidelines* to include a term for resting metabolism. The equation is now virtually identical to the original equation established by researchers in 1965 (Nagle, Balke, and Naughton, 1965). The oxygen cost for lifting one's body mass up the step is 1.8 ml for each kg · m of work (as in the walking and leg cycling equations). However, one-third must be added to account for the oxygen cost of eccentrically lowering the body mass back down. Thus, the equation on page 50 uses a factor of 2.4; that is, 1.8 + (1/3 of 1.8).

The stepping rate in the equation refers to complete four-cycle steps per minute: (1) Lift the first leg onto the bench; (2) step up and place the second leg on the bench; (3) step down with the first leg; (4) step down with the second leg. There are four movements making up one "step," so set your metronome at four times the desired stepping rate to help your clients stay on cadence. The first leg is doing all of the concentric (lifting) work and the second leg is doing all the eccentric (lowering) work, so instruct clients to switch legs occasionally. They can do this by tapping the second leg on the floor at the end of a cycle and immediately lifting it back onto the step.

CASE STUDY 4.9

Stepping—Solve for the $\dot{V}O_2$

Kathy is a 46-year-old aerobic dance instructor. During her stepping classes, she leads her clients in a routine performed at 20 steps per minute (to a beat of 80 min⁻¹). If the class is using 4 in. benches, what is their estimated $\dot{V}O_2$ in ml · min⁻¹ · kg⁻¹ and in METs?

First, convert terms. The step height must be entered into the equation in meters. One inch is equal to 2.54 cm, or to 0.0254 m.

$$4 \text{ in.} \times 0.0254 = 0.10 \text{ m}$$

Second, select the stepping equation from page 50, enter the known values, and solve for the unknown $\dot{V}O_2$:

$\dot{V}O_2 = 3.5 + 0.2(\text{stepping rate}) + 2.4(\text{stepping rate})(\text{step height})$

$\quad = 3.5 + 0.2(20) + 2.4(20)(0.10)$

$\quad = 3.5 + 4.0 + 4.8$

$\quad = 12.3 \text{ ml} \cdot \text{min}^{-1} \cdot \text{kg}^{-1}$ *(continued)*

Case Study 4.9   *(continued)*

Third, convert to the desired units.

$$(12.3 \text{ ml} \cdot \text{min}^{-1} \cdot \text{kg}^{-1}) / 3.5 = 3.5 \text{ METs}$$

CASE STUDY 4.10

Stepping—Solve for the Workload

One member of Kathy's stepping class, Tasha, has purchased a set of stackable benches for use at home. The benches come in 2 in. increments and can be stacked to a height of 10 in. Tasha is 32 years old, weighs 128 lb, and is in the low-risk category. Her $\dot{V}O_2$max has been estimated as 38 ml $\cdot$ min^{-1} $\cdot$ kg^{-1}. To exercise at 70% of $\dot{V}O_2R$, what stepping rate would she need on the 10 in. bench? At what rate should she set her metronome?

First, convert the bench height to meters and determine the target $\dot{V}O_2$ from the $\dot{V}O_2R$ formula:

$$10 \text{ in.} \times 0.0254 = 0.254 \text{ m}$$

$$\text{Target } \dot{V}O_2 = (\text{intensity fraction})(\dot{V}O_2\text{max} - 3.5) + 3.5$$

$$= (0.70)(38 - 3.5) + 3.5$$

$$= (0.70)(34.5) + 3.5$$

$$= 24.15 + 3.5$$

$$= 27.7 \text{ ml} \cdot \text{min}^{-1} \cdot \text{kg}^{-1}$$

Second, select the stepping equation from page 50, enter the known values, and solve for the unknown stepping rate:

$\dot{V}O_2 = 3.5 + 0.2(\text{stepping rate}) + 2.4(\text{stepping rate})(\text{step height})$

$27.7 = 3.5 + 0.2(\text{stepping rate}) + 2.4(\text{stepping rate})(0.254)$

$27.7 = 3.5 + 0.2(\text{stepping rate}) + 0.6096(\text{stepping rate})$

$27.7 = 3.5 + (0.2 + 0.6096)(\text{stepping rate})$

$27.7 = 3.5 + 0.8096(\text{stepping rate})$

$27.7 - 3.5 = 0.8096(\text{stepping rate})$

$24.2 = 0.8096(\text{stepping rate})$

$24.2/0.8096 = \text{stepping rate}$

$29.89 \text{ steps} \cdot \text{min}^{-1} = \text{stepping rate}$

The stepping rate for Tasha should be 30 steps per minute. She should set her metronome at four times this, or 120 min^{-1}.

REFERENCES

ACSM. 2006. *ACSM's Guidelines for Exercise Testing and Prescription*, 7th ed., 286-299. Philadelphia: Lippincott Williams & Wilkins.

Bassett, D.R., M.D. Giese, F.J. Nagle, A. Ward, D.M. Raab, and B. Balke.1985. Aerobic requirements of overground versus treadmill running. *Medicine and Science in Sports and Exercise* 17: 477-481.

Franklin, B.A. 1985. Exercise testing, training and arm ergometry. *Sports Medicine* 2: 100-119.

Lang, P.B., R.W. Latin, K.E. Berg, and M.B. Mellion. 1992. The accuracy of the ACSM cycle ergometry equation. *Medicine and Science in Sports and Exercise* 24: 272-276.

Latin, R.W., and K.E. Berg. 1994. The accuracy of the ACSM and a new cycle ergometry equation for young women. *Medicine and Science in Sports and Exercise* 26: 642-646.

Londeree, B.R., J. Moffitt-Gerstenberger, J.A. Padfield, and D. Lottmann.1997. Oxygen consumption of cycle ergometry is nonlinearly related to work rate and pedal rate. *Medicine and Science in Sports and Exercise* 29: 775-780.

Minetti, A.E., C. Moia, G.S. Roi, D. Susta, and G. Ferretti. 2002. Energy cost of walking and running at extreme uphill and downhill slopes. *Journal of Applied Physiology* 93: 1039-1046.

Nagle, F.J., B. Balke, and J.P. Naughton. 1965. Gradational step tests for assessing work capacity. *Journal of Applied Physiology* 20: 745-748.

Swain, D.P. 2000. Energy cost calculations for exercise prescription: An update. *Sports Medicine* 30: 17-22.

5

Exercise Prescription
for Weight Loss

Obesity is a major risk factor for chronic disease, and it results in substantial health care costs. Currently, obesity continues to increase in Americans across all sociodemographic groups and in all parts of the United States. The most recent National Health and Nutrition Examination Survey, NHANES III, reported that 31% of Americans are obese, with a total of 65% being either overweight or obese (Flegal et al., 2002). Increased incidence of obesity is accompanied by an increase in diabetes. According to NHANES III, 9% of U.S. adults have diabetes and another 26% have the prediabetic condition of impaired fasting glucose (Cowie et al., 2006). Most experts recognize that the prevalence of obesity is likely to increase in the future.

Obesity may or may not be a health risk itself. However, when body fat percentages exceed 25% and 30% in sedentary males and females, respectively, or body mass index exceeds 30 kg · m^{-2}, the risk for hypokinetic diseases—such as heart disease, high blood pressure, and diabetes— increases. Furthermore, even with all the low-fat and nonfat food choices, this percentage is increasing as advancing technology creates a more sedentary society. Although exercise can play an important role in combating obesity, compliance is a significant problem. Among sedentary adults who begin an exercise program, 50% drop out within the first three to six months (ACSM, 2006b).

ENERGY BALANCE

People gain weight when they achieve a positive caloric balance—that is, when they consume more calories than they expend. Figure 5.1 illustrates various sources of energy intake and energy expenditure. Energy intake is approximately 4 kcal per gram of carbohydrates or protein, 7 kcal per gram of ethyl alcohol, and 9 kcal per gram of fat. The actual energy values for these chemical substances are somewhat higher, but the amount absorbed by the body is less than the amount actually eaten; and in the case of proteins, a portion of the caloric value is lost when amino acids are deaminated for caloric use.

Energy expenditure is due to resting metabolic rate (RMR), the thermic effect of food, and muscular activity. **Resting metabolic rate** is approximately 1 kcal per hour for each kilogram of body mass. However, it is lower for people with a high proportion of body fat, because adipose tissue has a lower metabolic rate than

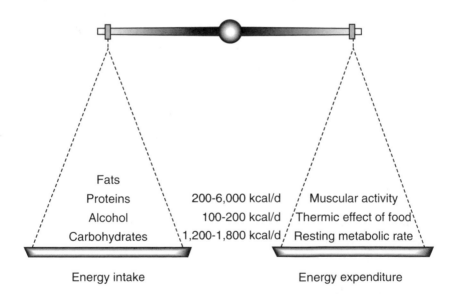

Fats		
Proteins	200-6,000 kcal/d	Muscular activity
Alcohol	100-200 kcal/d	Thermic effect of food
Carbohydrates	1,200-1,800 kcal/d	Resting metabolic rate

Energy intake   Energy expenditure

Figure 5.1   Energy balance is determined by caloric intake from various food sources versus energy expenditure. Resting metabolic rate and the thermic effect of food are relatively fixed values, but energy expenditure from muscular activity varies tremendously based on an individual's personal choices. If energy expenditure exceeds intake, weight loss will occur.

does lean tissue. The digestion and assimilation of food is an energy-requiring process known as the **thermic effect of food,** and it expends 5 to 10% of the calories consumed. The most variable source of energy expenditure is muscular activity. Sedentary people may expend no more than 200 to 300 kcal per day in activities of daily living, and people with physically demanding jobs or who engage in structured exercise might expend several hundred, and up to a few thousand, additional kcal per day. Competitors in the Tour de France bicycle race need to consume 6,000 to 8,000 kcal per day to maintain caloric balance (Saris et al., 1989).

If a person is in a positive energy balance, the excess calories will be stored in the body. Carbohydrates can be stored as glycogen, but total body stores of glycogen are only 1,000 to 2,000 kcal. Once glycogen stores are filled, any excessive carbohydrate consumption will be converted to fat and stored as adipose tissue. Proteins can be "stored" as muscle tissue but only if the person is engaged in a properly structured resistance training program. Even then, the rate of muscular growth is very slow, especially in highly trained subjects, being only a few pounds per year under the best conditions. Therefore, most protein intake that exceeds daily needs is converted to fat and stored as adipose tissue. Any alcohol or fat that is consumed in excess of immediate caloric needs is also stored as adipose tissue. The body is well designed to store any source of excess calories as fat, as a protection against famine. In modern society, this storage of fat is generally unnecessary and is clearly not worth the risk of associated chronic diseases.

WEIGHT MANAGEMENT

Body composition can be measured by a variety of methods, some of which are better than others. For example, methods that distinguish between body fat and lean muscle are regarded as the best because a person can be overweight without being overfat. A very athletic or muscular person, for instance, might fall into the overweight category.

A specific cause for obesity is yet to be discovered. It appears to be multifactorial in nature, with inactivity being a leading component. Therefore, therapy should address behavioral, social, and cultural factors. Long-term medications for the treatment of obesity are not available. Current medications include sympatho-mimetics and serotonin inhibitors. These medications appear to result in weight loss, yet for safety concerns, their long-term use is not recommended. Moreover, weight gain usually returns when the medications are discontinued. Unfortunately, the failure or recidivism rate for weight loss programs is approximately 70 to 95% (Leutholtz and Ripoll, 1999).

The exercise prescription for an obese client should encourage overall energy expenditure that can be maintained to achieve long-term weight management. To accomplish this, the four variables of the FITT principle (as outlined in chapter 3) should be followed. The primary mode or type of exercise should include activities that target large muscle groups. To maximize caloric expenditure, the intensity should be low to moderate (e.g., 40 to 60% $\dot{V}O_2R$ or HRR). This will allow more emphasis to be placed on the duration and frequency of exercise, which may be from 45 to 60 minutes a day, five to seven days per week (ACSM, 2006a). Intensity can be increased to 50 to 75% of the $\dot{V}O_2R$ or HRR as tolerated, in conjunction with adjustments in the duration.

The volume of exercise, which is the product of the intensity and duration, should amount to a minimum of 2,000 kcal per week accomplished within three to five hours.

For example, in the exercise prescriptions, you should emphasize duration and frequency (progressing to one hour daily) over intensity until your client can exercise at an intensity suitable for cardiovascular conditioning. You should also instruct your client in proper eating habits; that is, consuming a well-balanced diet that is low in fat and moderately reduced in total calories.

EXERCISE PRESCRIPTION FOR FAT LOSS

In designing exercise prescriptions for reducing body fat, always consider the four basic variables of aerobic exercise—frequency, intensity, time (duration), and type of exercise (the FITT formula). Once your client has settled into a regular program of aerobic exercise, you can add weightlifting to the program. However, the initial focus should be on increasing the volume of exercise and caloric expenditure, which can best be achieved by doing aerobic exercise. Resistance training can result in a small increase in lean body mass, which will increase caloric expenditure by increasing resting metabolism, but this effect is comparatively small.

An important consideration in prescribing exercise is to recognize that only the *net* caloric expenditure can be counted toward fat loss. The net caloric expenditure is that which is due to the exercise itself, whereas the gross caloric expenditure is the net value plus the amount associated with rest. The resting caloric expenditure should not be counted toward fat loss (unless the client is fasting), because the client would burn those same calories whether or not he or she was exercising.

Exercise is critical for properly achieving a negative caloric balance. However, sedentary people are not capable of performing at a high rate of energy expenditure, and thus must accumulate a large total duration on a weekly basis to effectively lose fat weight. For example, walking at 3.5 mph (about a 17-minute-per-mile pace) burns only 3.3 kcal per minute above resting energy expenditure for a 70 kg (154 lb) client (a heavier client would burn proportionally more). If the same person could run at 7 mph (about an 8 1/2-minute-per-mile pace), he or she would burn calories four times faster. For each mile covered, the runner burns twice as many calories as the walker and is covering miles twice as fast, thus accounting for the fourfold greater rate of expenditure.

A common error is to assume that walking and running burn the same number of calories per mile, often estimated as 100 kcal. However, this refers to the *gross* number of calories, including those due to resting metabolism. Because walkers take longer to cover the mile, they burn more calories associated with the resting component than runners do, resulting in similar totals per mile. For weight loss purposes, however, only the net caloric expenditure can be counted. As figure 5.2 illustrates, walkers would need a little over an hour of exercise seven days per week to lose 1/2 lb of fat, whereas runners would obtain as much weight loss with only 30 minutes of exercise, four days a week.

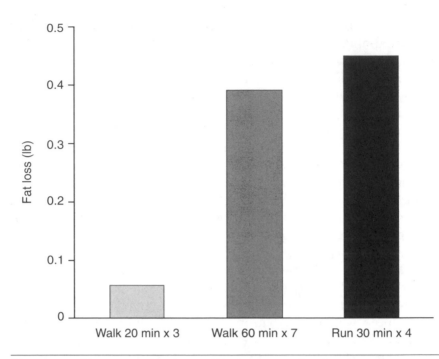

Figure 5.2   The amount of fat that would be lost by exercise alone (assuming no increase in caloric consumption) by a 154 lb (70 kg) person. Fat loss by heavier people would be proportionally greater. "Walking" is at 3.5 mph, burning a net 3.3 kcal per minute. "Running" is at 7.0 mph, burning a net 13.1 kcal per minute.

CASE STUDY 5.1

Weight Loss Client

Arthur is a sedentary 40-year-old man who has been gradually gaining weight for the last 10 years. He recently saw his medical doctor for a routine physical. His current weight and height are 250 lb and 5'9". His body mass index is 37 kg · m^{-2}. He reported that he was experiencing chest pain and stated that his brother had a heart attack when he was 47. His physician performed a maximal cardiopulmonary stress test and obtained the following results: $\dot{V}O_2$max of 30 ml · min^{-1} · kg^{-1}, maximal HR of 170 bpm, resting HR of 90 bpm, normal ECG response to exercise, and no signs or symptoms of heart disease. His physician advised him to begin a weight loss program with an initial loss of 50 lb, and he referred him to you to begin an exercise program.

Arthur's goal weight is 200 lb. He is very anxious to lose weight and wants to reach his goal in just one month. However, you remind him that it has taken him 10 years to gain this weight, and a loss of 2 lb per week would result in a safer and more permanent reduction in about six months. You decide that stepping exercises and jogging are too rigorous for a sedentary overweight person. After discussing the other options with Arthur, you both agree that the best type of exercise for him is walking and stationary cycling. You ask him to begin with 20 to 30 minutes of walking every other day and to gradually increase this to at least 45 minutes on a daily basis.

Because Arthur has been sedentary for the last 10 years, you choose a fairly low to moderate window for his intensity—perhaps 50 to 70% of HRR, or $\dot{V}O_2R$. Because Arthur had a maximal stress test, in your calculations you can use his measured maximum HR of 170 bpm. Calculate a target heart rate at 50% and 70% of Arthur's HRR.

$$\text{Target HR} = (\text{intensity fraction})(\text{HRmax} - \text{HRrest}) + \text{HRrest}$$

$$\text{Lower target HR} = (0.5)(170 - 90) + 90$$

$$= (0.5)(80) + 90$$

$$= 40 + 90$$

$$= 130 \text{ bpm}$$

$$\text{Upper target HR} = (0.7)(170 - 90) + 90$$

$$= (0.7)(80) + 90$$

$$= 56 + 90$$

$$= 146 \text{ bpm}$$

Next, Arthur tells you that he has to walk a brisk 3.7 mph on a treadmill at 0% grade to reach the lower end of his heart rate prescription of 130 bpm. How many calories is he burning at this point? To determine this, first calculate his $\dot{V}O_2$ using the walking equation from page 50. Table 4.1 indicates that, to convert mph to m · min^{-1}, multiply by 26.8. Thus, the speed is 3.7 mph × 26.8 = 99.2 m · min^{-1}.

(continued)

Case Study 5.1 *(continued)*

$$\dot{V}O_2 = 3.5 + 0.1(\text{speed}) + 1.8(\text{speed})(\text{fractional grade})$$

$$= 3.5 + 0.1(99.2) + 1.8(99.2)(0)$$

$$= 3.5 + 9.92 + 0$$

$$= 13.4 \text{ ml} \cdot \text{min}^{-1} \cdot \text{kg}^{-1} \text{ (gross } \dot{V}O_2)$$

$$\text{Net } \dot{V}O_2 = 13.4 - 3.5 = 9.9 \text{ ml} \cdot \text{min}^{-1} \cdot \text{kg}^{-1}$$

(Note that this is less than 50% of his $\dot{V}O_2R$. This workload was chosen on the basis of his target HR, and target HRs and target $\dot{V}O_2$s will not always match because both are estimates of his actual physiological responses.)

Now, convert to caloric expenditure by using the conversion formulas in table 4.2. First, convert $\dot{V}O_2$ in ml $\cdot$ min$^{-1}\cdot$ kg^{-1} to L $\cdot$ min^{-1}; then convert the $\dot{V}O_2$ to kcal $\cdot$ min^{-1}.

$$\frac{(9.9 \text{ ml} \cdot \text{min}^{-1} \cdot \text{kg}^{-1})(113.6 \text{ kg})}{1,000} = 1.12 \text{ L} \cdot \text{min}^{-1}$$

Next, remember that 5 kcal are expended for each liter of oxygen consumed; therefore, during a 45-minute exercise session, Arthur would burn the following number of calories:

$$(1.12 \text{ L} \cdot \text{min}^{-1}) \times 5 = 5.6 \text{ kcal} \cdot \text{min}^{-1}$$

(5.6 kcal $\cdot$ min^{-1}) $\times$ (45 min) $= 252$ kcal per a 45-minute exercise session

Finally, do one more calculation with Arthur. Three months have passed, and as a result of Arthur's exercise and dietary changes, he has lost 25 lb and is now able to jog and achieve the upper end of his target heart rate range, 146 bpm. To achieve this heart rate he tells you that he must now jog at 4.5 mph. He has not been able to increase his exercise session from 45 minutes but wants to know how many calories he is burning. To calculate this figure, use the running equation from page 50. His speed is 4.5 mph $\times$ 26.8 $= 120.6$ m $\cdot$ min^{-1}.

$$\dot{V}O_2 = 3.5 + 0.2(\text{speed}) + 0.9(\text{speed})(\text{fractional grade})$$

$$\dot{V}O_2 = 3.5 + 0.2(120.6) + 0.9(120.6)(0)$$

$$= 3.5 + 24.12 + 0$$

$$\dot{V}O_2 = 27.6 \text{ ml} \cdot \text{min}^{-1} \cdot \text{kg}^{-1} \text{ (gross } \dot{V}O_2)$$

$$\text{Net } \dot{V}O_2 = 27.6 - 3.5 = 24.1 \text{ ml} \cdot \text{min}^{-1} \cdot \text{kg}^{-1}$$

(Note that this is more than 70% of $\dot{V}O_2R$ based on his original $\dot{V}O_2$max. However, his aerobic capacity has improved and, as noted earlier, his workloads based on HR and based on $\dot{V}O_2$ will not match precisely.)

Convert to $L \cdot min^{-1}$ and then to kcal $\cdot min^{-1}$. Note that his new body mass is 225 lb/2.2 = 102.3 kg:

$$\frac{(24.1 \text{ ml} \cdot min^{-1} \cdot kg^{-1}) \times (102.3 \text{ kg})}{1,000} = 2.47 \text{ L} \cdot min^{-1}$$

$$(2.47 \text{ L} \cdot min^{-1}) \times 5 = 12.3 \text{ kcal} \cdot min^{-1}$$

$$(12.3 \text{ kcal} \cdot min^{-1}) \times (45 \text{ minutes}) = 554 \text{ kcal}$$
for each 45-minute exercise session

Arthur has doubled his caloric expenditure by increasing his intensity or speed.

Arthur's exercise prescription can be summarized as follows:

Frequency: A minimum of five days per week to maximize caloric expenditure.

Intensity: A target heart rate range of 130 to 146 beats per minute, to place him at approximately 50 to 70% of $\dot{V}O_2R$. (If a person is not able to maintain a target heart rate continuously, the intensity should be decreased and the time increased to maintain caloric expenditure.)

Time: Arthur requires at least 45 minutes of exercise to achieve the recommended 300 to 500 kcal expenditure per exercise session.

Type: You have prescribed modalities that exercise large muscle groups, such as walking and cycling, to maximize caloric expenditure. (Note that non-weight-bearing activities are recommended for people with orthopedic concerns.)

CASE STUDY 5.2
Weight Loss Client

Another client, Sheila, is obese with a body fat percentage of 37%, measured by the underwater weighing, or hydrodensitometry, method. Her current weight is 205 lb, she is 5'5" tall, and her age is 32. Her body mass index (BMI) is 34 kg $\cdot m^{-2}$. Sheila has osteoarthritis but does not have a significant history of, or risk factors for, heart disease. She has been referred to you by her physician for an exercise program designed to help her lose weight.

(continued)

Case Study 5.2   *(continued)*

Because Sheila has two ACSM risk factors—obesity and sedentary behavior—she is in the moderate-risk category. Yet she already
has her physician's recommendation that she exercise. As a starting
point, she agrees to a goal of reaching 30% fat. To determine her
goal weight at this level, use the following formula. In the formula,
% fat must be entered as a fraction.

$$\text{Goal weight} = \frac{(\text{current weight})(1 - \text{current \% fat})}{(1 - \text{desired \% fat})}$$

$$\text{Goal weight} = (205)(1 - 0.37) / (1 - 0.30)$$

$$= (205)(0.63) / (0.70)$$

$= 129 / 0.70$ (i.e., her lean body weight is 129
lb, and you would like this to be 70% of her
total, instead of 63%)

$$= 184 \text{ lb}$$

Now that you have determined an initial goal weight for Sheila,
develop her exercise prescription. Because of her arthritis, a stationary bike might be a good choice for the mode of exercise. She
agrees to exercise at least five days per week and to gradually
increase her duration to one hour per session. You have decided
to set the intensity level at 50% to 75% of $\dot{V}O_2R$, using the %HRR
method. Having instructed Sheila to take her resting heart rate when
she wakes up in the morning, you estimate her maximal heart rate
using the calculation 220 – age. Her resting heart rate is reported
to be 85 bpm, and her estimated maximal heart rate is 220 – 32 =
188 bpm. Now calculate her target heart rate range:

$$\text{Target HR} = (\text{intensity fraction})(\text{HRmax} - \text{HRrest}) + \text{HRrest}$$

$$\text{Lower target HR} = (0.5)(188 - 85) + 85$$

$$= (0.5)(103) + 85$$

$$= 51.5 + 85$$

$$= 136 \text{ bpm}$$

$$\text{Upper target HR} = (0.7)(188 - 85) + 85$$

$$= (0.7)(103) + 85$$

$$= 72 + 85$$

$$= 157 \text{ bpm}$$

Sheila tells you that to exercise in her heart rate range of 136 to 157 bpm, she must pedal her stationary bike at 75 W or 450 kg · m · min^{-1} (1 W is approximately equal to 6 kg · m · min^{-1}). First calculate her $\dot{V}O_2$ at this intensity using the cycling equation from page 50.

$$\dot{V}O_2 = 7 + 1.8(\text{work rate}) / (\text{body mass})$$

$$= 7 + 1.8(450)/93.2$$

$$= 7 + 810/93.2$$

$$= 7 + 8.7$$

$$= 15.7 \text{ ml} \cdot \text{min}^{-1} \cdot \text{kg}^{-1} \text{ (gross } \dot{V}O_2)$$

$$\text{Net } \dot{V}O_2 = 15.7 - 3.5 = 12.2 \text{ ml} \cdot \text{min}^{-1} \cdot \text{kg}^{-1}$$

Convert your answer to liters per minute and multiply by 5 to calculate how many kcal Sheila is expending per minute of exercise (remember to use *net* $\dot{V}O_2$).

$$\frac{(12.2 \text{ ml} \cdot \text{min}^{-1} \cdot \text{kg}^{-1}) \ (93.2 \text{ kg})}{1,000} = 1.14 \text{ L} \cdot \text{min}^{-1}$$

$$(1.14 \text{ L} \cdot \text{min}^{-1}) \times 5 = 5.7 \text{ kcal} \cdot \text{min}^{-1}$$

$$(5.7 \text{ kcal} \cdot \text{min}^{-1}) \times (60 \text{ min}) = 342 \text{ kcal per}$$
$$\text{a 60-minute exercise session}$$

Sheila has a current weight of 205 lb and a goal weight of 184 lb, for a total weight loss of 21 lb. Remind her that an appropriate amount of weight to lose is no more than 1 kg per week, or approximately 2 lb. At that rate, it will take Sheila about 10 weeks to reach her goal weight. If she exercised five days per week for 60 minutes, she would expend $342 \times 5 = 1,710$ *net* kcal per week

(continued)

Case Study 5.2   *(continued)*

as a result of exercise. However, remember that 2 lb of fat contains 7,000 kcal. Therefore, to lose 2 lb per week, the remaining 5,290 kcal reduction each week (or 5,290 / 7 = 756 kcal per day) should come from a modification in her diet. You might consider recommending that Sheila consult a registered dietitian.

REFERENCES

ACSM. 2006a. *ACSM's Guidelines for Exercise Testing and Prescription,* 7th ed., 216-219. Philadelphia: Lippincott Williams & Wilkins.

ACSM. 2006b. *ACSM's Resource Manual for Guidelines for Exercise Testing and Prescription,* 5th ed., 565. Philadelphia: Lippincott Williams and Wilkins.

Cowie, C.C., K.F. Rust, D.D. Byrd-Holt, et al. 2006. Prevalence of diabetes and impaired fasting glucose in adults in the U.S. population: National Health and Nutrition Examination Survey 1999-2002. *Diabetes Care* 29: 1263-1268.

Flegal, K.M., M.D. Carroll, B. Goodpaster, et al. 2002. Prevalence and trends in obesity among U.S. adults, 1999-2000. *Journal of the American Medical Association* 288: 1723-1727.

Leutholtz, B.C., and I. Ripoll. 1999. *Exercise and Disease Management,* ed. I. Wolinsky, 97-104. Boca Raton, FL: CRC Press.

Saris, W.H.M., M.A. van Erp-Baart, F. Brouns, K.R., 1989. Westerterp, and F. tenHoor. Study on food intake and energy expenditure during extreme sustained exercise. The Tour de France. *International Journal of Sports Medicine* 10: 526-531.

CHAPTER

6

Exercise Prescription
for Flexibility
and Muscular Strength

What defines a "fit" person? If this question were asked back in the early 1900s, the answer might have been "someone who can chop a cord of wood." The answer in the 1940s might have been "an individual with huge muscles, like Charles Atlas." In the 1970s one might have answered, "someone who, like my neighbor, runs every morning and competes in weekend marathons." The definition of fitness has evolved over the past century. Today, being fit only aerobically or only in terms in muscle strength does not account for overall fitness. People should strive for optimum function in all components of fitness to achieve total body health. This chapter focuses on resistance training and flexibility guidelines as part of total fitness.

FLEXIBILITY

Flexibility involves moving a joint through its entire range of motion. Having good flexibility is important not only in athletic performance but also in everyday activities. All exercise programs should include exercises that promote the improvement or maintenance of flexibility. Lack of flexibility is associated with back pain and a reduced ability to perform activities of daily living.

When to Stretch

Stretching, a very important part of an exercise prescription, is often neglected or performed improperly. Ideally, stretching should be done when the core temperature of the muscle is sufficiently warmed up. For warming to occur, the muscle must be actively contracted. Although sitting in the sun or in a hot tub may make you feel warm because the core temperature of your body rises, this does not properly warm up the skeletal muscles in preparation for exercise. The safest time to stretch is during the cool-down following an aerobic or resistance exercise session, when the muscles are still warm. However, stretching also may be included at the end of the warm-up to an exercise session, or at a separate time as long as a specific warm-up is performed for the stretching session itself.

Flexibility in the lower-back and posterior thigh regions is particularly important to decrease the risk of lower-back injuries and pain. A regular stretching program may reduce the decline in flexibility that occurs with aging, and it may improve balance, especially in older adults. Because flexibility is joint specific, no single stretch will result in total body flexibility.

Types of Stretches

There are three different types of stretches—static, ballistic, and proprioceptive neuromuscular facilitation (PNF). *Static stretches are the preferred method for most people to maintain or improve range of motion in a joint.* The risk of injury is lowest with static stretches, and they require little time and assistance to be effective.

How to Stretch

In **static stretching,** the muscle group is slowly stretched to the point of tension or mild discomfort and held for 15 to 30 seconds. Each stretch should be performed two to four times. This combination of duration and frequency recommended by the ACSM is appropriate for obtaining some improvement in flexibility. For optimum results, however, each stretch should be held for a minute or longer. The ACSM-recommended frequency of stretching is at least two days per week and preferably five to seven days per week (ACSM, 2006). See figures 6.1 through 6.5 for examples of static stretches.

The second type of stretch is the ballistic stretch. The **ballistic stretch** is a "dynamic" stretch because it involves active, bouncing movements. If this stretch is performed too aggressively or the joint's range of motion is exceeded, it can injure the connective tissue. Furthermore, if the muscle is suddenly stretched very forcefully, a reflex contraction may occur that can actually shorten the muscle and inhibit the stretch. The ballistic stretch may have a place in the warm-up, *provided the types of movements performed during the workout are similar to the stretch;* however, the ACSM does not recommend the use of the ballistic stretch.

The final type of stretch is **proprioceptive neuromuscular facilitation,** or the **PNF stretch.** The PNF stretch has been reported to produce the greatest improvements in flexibility (Pollock et al., 1998). However, it can cause muscle soreness. The PNF stretch involves contracting and relaxing opposing muscle groups with the assistance of a partner. An example of a PNF stretch for the hamstring is as follows: The client lies on his back on a table and lifts one leg into the air. A partner places his shoulder under the client's calf and gently pushes the client's leg to the end of its range of motion. Next, the client pushes down against the partner's shoulder with his leg to forcefully contract his hamstrings and gluteals. This contraction is held for six seconds. At the moment the client ceases the contraction, the partner pushes the leg farther up, resulting in a greater stretch of the muscles. This stretch can be further enhanced through the process of **reciprocal inhibition,** in which the client forcefully contracts the antagonist muscles, in this case the quadriceps, during the stretch. Like static stretches, PNF stretches should be held for 15 to 30 seconds, performed two to four times, and be done at least two times per week.

Figures 6.1 through 6.5 provide some examples of static stretches. For a more comprehensive listing of stretching exercises, see the National Strength and Conditioning Association's second edition of *Essentials of Strength Training and Conditioning* (Baechle and Earle, 2000).

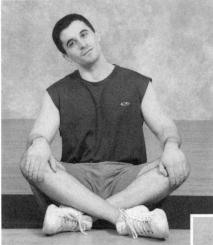

◄ **Figure 6.1** Neck stretch (muscles of the neck). Gently move your head from side to side so that your ear moves toward your shoulder. Then move your head forward and back so that your chin drops down toward your chest and then return your head to a vertical position. Do not hyperextend your neck back or do complete circles in a rapid motion.

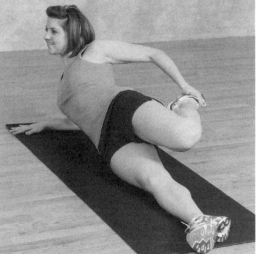

Figure 6.2 Quadriceps stretch (muscles of the anterior thigh). Gently pull your ankle toward your gluteals. When you feel tension, hold. Avoid pulling your heel tight against your gluteals; rather, pull your entire leg back. ►

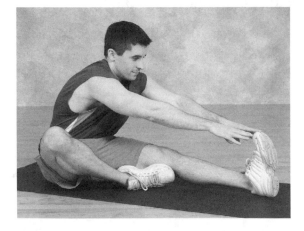

◄ **Figure 6.3** Hamstring stretch (muscles of the posterior thigh). In a seated position with one leg extended, bend the other leg so that the sole of the foot rests against the inside of the extended leg's thigh or knee. Begin with an upright torso and lean forward without curving the back. Grasp the extended leg or foot to pull the torso further forward.

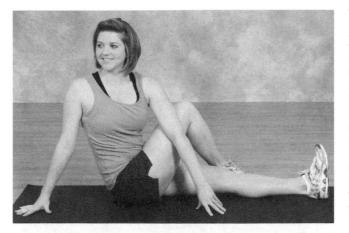

◀ **Figure 6.4**   Sit-and-twist (muscles of the trunk and back). Sitting on the floor, bend your right leg and cross it over your left leg. Place your left elbow across your body outside your right knee and your right hand on the floor behind you; slowly rotate to the right and then hold. Repeat for the opposite side.

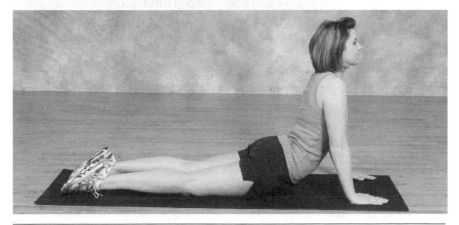

▲ **Figure 6.5**   Back hypertension stretch (muscles of the lower back and abdomen). Lie prone on the floor. With your arms extended and palms flat on the floor, slowly arch your chest and hold. Do not push your hips up off the floor.

MUSCULAR STRENGTH

Muscular strength refers to the greatest force that can be generated by a specific muscle group or groups. It can be measured by a variety of devices such as handgrip dynamometers and cable tensiometers, or by performing or estimating a one-repetition maximum (1RM). **Muscular endurance** is the ability to perform multiple repetitions at a given percentage of 1RM. People with a high degree of muscular strength can perform activities of daily living, as well as athletic pursuits, at lower percentages of 1RM, and thus with less relative effort.

Resistance Training Guidelines

The major benefits of resistance training include maintaining or increasing muscular strength and endurance, muscle mass, bone density, and metabolic rate. Skeletal muscles adapt or improve in size and strength when an overload is applied. This overload can be accomplished by increasing the **intensity** (i.e., the resistance or weight), **duration** (number of sets performed), or **frequency** of the workouts. One complete repetition of a lift involves two phases. First is the **concentric** phase, when the muscle shortens as it applies force to lift the weight. Second is the **eccentric** phase, when the weight is returned to its starting position. During the eccentric phase, the muscle is still applying force, but it is being lengthened. Dynamic resistance programs that include both concentric and eccentric components are of the greatest benefit. Routines that emphasize the eccentric component may increase muscle soreness.

The number of repetitions to fatigue determines the *intensity* of resistance exercise. Lifting a weight that fatigues the muscle after 8 to 12 repetitions develops muscular strength *and* endurance. For most exercises, this number of repetitions can be done with a weight that is approximately 80% of the maximal lift (i.e., 80% of the one-repetition maximum, or 1RM). The greatest increases in strength occur when a person lifts heavier weights that produce fatigue with fewer than 8 repetitions. To build muscular endurance, however, one should use lighter weights and more than 12 repetitions per set (Pollock et al., 1998). Thus, the 8- to 12RM range is a compromise intended to improve both strength and muscular endurance. To focus more on strength, a 3- to 8RM range should be used, and to focus more on muscular endurance, a 13- to 20RM range should be used (ACSM, 2006).

You can determine the weight that represents 8- to 12RM for a client in two ways. One way is simply trial and error. Begin with a very light weight and ask the client to perform 12 repetitions. If she can do this without complete fatigue on the last repetition, increase the weight until she can perform at least 8 repetitions but no more than 12. Alternatively, you can determine the 1RM (also by trial and error) and then use 80% of this value in the first training session. If this weight causes fatigue in fewer than 8 repetitions, reduce it; if your client can perform more than 12 repetitions with this weight, increase it. Continue to adjust the weight until fatigue occurs within the 8- to 12-repetition range. Once the 8- to 12RM is established by either technique, clients enter the progressive phase of training in which the weight is increased by about 10% whenever they reach 12 repetitions.

The *time*, or duration, of a resistance training workout depends on the number of exercises performed and the number of sets performed for each exercise. The ACSM recommends that beginning lifters perform 8 to 10 different exercises that train all of the major muscle groups in a single exercise session. At least one set of each exercise should be performed. Multiple sets may produce somewhat greater gains, but the total duration of the workout session should be no more than one hour. Longer sessions may result in client attrition.

The ACSM recommends a *frequency* of two or three resistance training sessions per week. These sessions should occur on alternate days, allowing at least 48 hours of recovery time between workouts. People who perform more advanced routines may use multiple sets and exercises for specific muscle groups; typically, they split the routine into two or more parts and perform each part only two days per week.

Resistance Training Technique

It is critical that you teach clients proper weightlifting technique to optimize strength gains and to ensure their safety.

The components of proper weightlifting form are full range of motion (ROM), isolation, controlled movement speed, and proper breathing.

- **Full range of motion.** Each lift should be performed through the greatest ROM available for the joint or joints being targeted by the exercise. Partial movements will result in adaptations specific to the limited range that was used.

- **Isolation.** Each lift should be performed so that only the target muscles contribute to the movement. Use of accessory muscles (so-called "cheating" movements) is common among lifters who are motivated solely to increase the weight. A greater training effect of the target muscles will occur when they are maximally stimulated and not assisted by other muscle groups. Examples of cheating are arching the back during a bench press and swaying the torso backward during a biceps curl.

• **Controlled movement speed.** The speed of movement throughout an exercise should be slow enough for the client to maintain control over the weight. Rapid concentric movement creates too much momentum and results in the muscle not being stimulated during the latter portion of the concentric action. Rapid eccentric movements ("dropping" the weight) deprive the muscle of stimulation during the eccentric phase and can also lead to injury. The ACSM recommends that each phase take approximately three seconds.

• **Proper breathing.** Proper breathing entails avoiding the Valsalva maneuver. Clients often perform a Valsalva maneuver (attempting to exhale against a closed glottis; i.e., "straining") during the concentric phase of the lift. This action significantly elevates arterial blood pressure, potentially damaging blood vessels (e.g., Valsalva retinopathy), and can provoke coronary ischemia in heart patients. If the Valsalva maneuver is held for an extended period of time, arterial blood pressure will fall as a result of impaired venous return, potentially causing fainting and injury. Teach clients to maintain a normal breathing pattern during the lift, such as by exhaling on exertion.

Spotting Technique

Anyone using free weights should have a trainer or lifting partner serve as a spotter to ensure safety. The principal roles of the spotter are as follows:

- Ensure that the bar is loaded with equal weight on both sides, secured by collars.
- Ensure that the lifter uses a balanced grip.
- Assist the lifter in removing the bar from the rack.
- Be prepared to assist the lifter if he or she loses balance or is unable to complete a repetition.
- Assist the lifter in returning the bar to the rack.

Many spotters assist lifters with virtually every repetition. This is not proper spotting, because it prevents the lifters from developing the confidence and the motor control to handle the weight on their own. Furthermore, this assistance makes it difficult for the spotter to determine the proper rate of progression for the lifter because the spotter doesn't learn the lifter's true ability. An exception occurs with the advanced lifting technique of performing only eccentric, or "negative," repetitions. During negative repetitions, the spotter assists the lifter with each concentric lifting of the weight, and then the lifter slowly returns the weight to the starting point. This technique greatly increases delayed-onset muscle soreness and should not be used with novice lifters. Another exception is the use of "forced" repetitions at the conclusion of a normal set. Once the lifter reaches fatigue performing unassisted repetitions, the spotter may help the lifter perform one or more additional repetitions to increase the overall stress of the workout. Finally, advanced lifters also may use isometric lifts to increase their strength at a particular angle during the repetition. This technique involves overloading the bar, lowering it to the desired angle, or "sticking point," and performing an isometric contraction for several seconds. A spotter assists with the placement and removal of the bar.

Figures 6.6 through 6.14 provide examples of exercises that can be performed using free weights or machines. For a more comprehensive listing of resistance training exercises, see the National Strength and Conditioning Association's second edition of *Essentials of Strength Training and Conditioning* (Baechle and Earle, 2000).

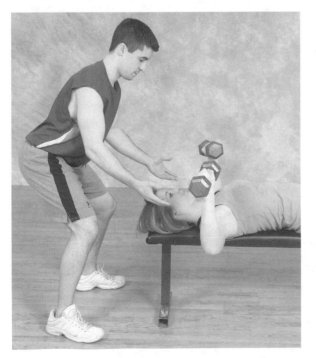

◄ **Figure 6.6** Bench press (muscles of the chest—pectorals; also anterior deltoids, triceps). Lying supine on a bench with your feet planted on the floor for balance, press the weight vertically until your arms are fully extended; then return the weight until the dumbbells (or bar) touch your chest. Your back and buttocks must remain in contact with the bench throughout the lift. Your spotter stands behind your head and bends at the hips and knees, keeping his back in a neutral position, to follow the path of the dumbbells. The spotter's hands are below the dumbbells, in preparation for assisting.

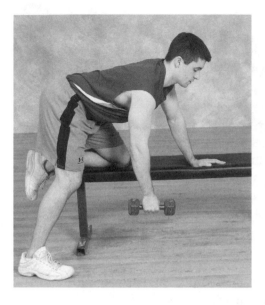

◀ **Figure 6.7** One-arm row (muscles of the back—latissimus dorsi, trapezius, rhomboids, teres major, biceps). Rest the left knee and left hand on a bench, keeping the left arm extended and the back flat. A dumbbell in the right hand is held directly below the right shoulder and lifted in a straight line toward the shoulder. Repeat on the other side.

Figure 6.8 Triceps extension (muscles of the posterior upper arm—triceps). From a standing position with the elbows held against the sides and the forearms approximately 30° above horizontal, press the bar downward to full extension; then return the bar to the starting position. Do not allow the bar to recover to a position higher than 30° above horizontal, which would cause the elbows to swing upward. ▶

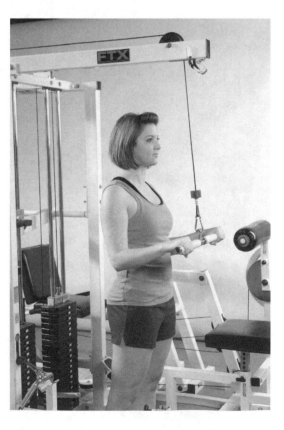

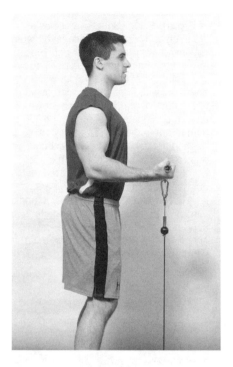

◀ **Figure 6.9** Biceps curl (muscles of the anterior upper arm—biceps, brachialis, brachioradialis). From a standing position, grasp the bar in an underhand (supinated) grip and stand erect with the elbows held firmly against the sides of your torso. Raise and lower the bar without swaying your back or moving the position of the elbows against the torso. This exercise may also be done in a seated position with back support, using dumbbells. From a seated position against back support, and with your elbows held against your sides, lift the dumbbells upward until your elbows are fully flexed; then return the weights to the fully extended position.

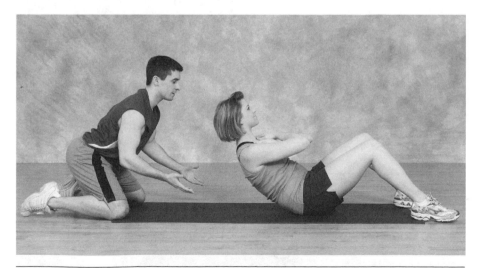

▲ **Figure 6.10** Curl-ups (abdominal muscles—rectus abdominis, obliques). Lying supine but with your knees bent at a 90° angle and your feet flat on the floor, curl your trunk upward until your shoulder blades are off the floor and your trunk reaches 30° above horizontal. Your arms are held across the shoulders, or, for less resistance, extended forward. A partner may support your head at the end of each repetition to avoid neck strain.

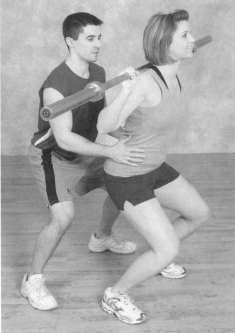

◄ Figure 6.11 Squats (muscles of the thigh and hips—quadriceps, gluteus maximus; also hamstrings, vasti, erector spinae). From a standing position with your feet at least shoulder-width apart and with the bar balanced on your upper back or shoulders, squat down until your thighs are parallel to the floor; then return to the standing position. Keep your head up to help maintain a relatively straight position of your back. Do not curve your back downward, and do not lower your thighs below parallel. Your spotter stands behind you and mimics your movement. Your spotter's hands are positioned along the sides and slightly in front of your chest to lift your torso if needed.

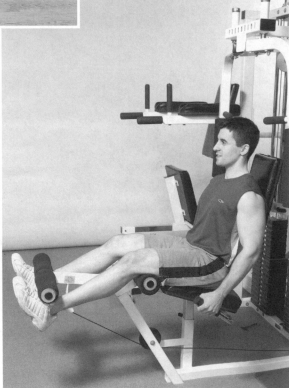

Figure 6.12 Leg extension (muscles of the anterior thigh—quadriceps). From a seated position with the back pad adjusted so that your knees are at the axis of rotation, and the ankle pad adjusted to just above your ankles, lift the weight to the full extension of your knees; then return to the starting position. ►

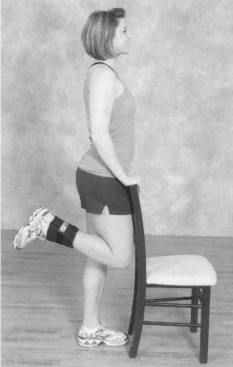

◄ **Figure 6.13** Leg curl (muscles of the posterior thigh—hamstrings). Place an ankle weight on one leg and stand behind a chair with your thighs touching the chair. Flex the knee to raise the leg as high as possible, without leaning your torso forward over the chair. This exercise may also be performed on a machine.

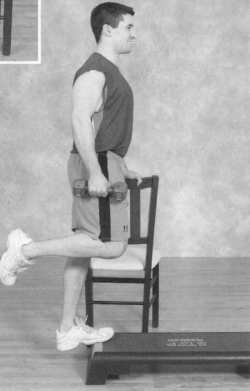

Figure 6.14 Calf raises (muscles of the posterior lower leg—gastrocnemius, soleus). From a standing position with one foot on an elevated surface, one hand holding a support for balance, and one hand holding a dumbbell, rise up on your toes as high as possible; then return to a position below parallel. Standing calf raises emphasize the gastrocnemius muscle, whereas seated calf raises, in which the knee is bent, emphasize the soleus muscle. ▶

Sedentary Client

Tanya is a 30-year-old, 145 lb (66 kg) female who is 5'4" (163 cm) tall (BMI of 24.9 kg · m^{-2}). She has decided that it is time to "get into shape" and "tone up." Tanya has not exercised aerobically since a high school physical education class and has never performed resistance training. She is a former cigarette smoker, having quit three months ago. She has no signs or symptoms of cardiopulmonary disease.

Tanya has two risk factors, sedentary behavior and cigarette smoking (she has to have quit for at least six months before we can discount that risk), placing her in the moderate-risk category. Therefore, she can begin a moderate-intensity exercise program without first seeking physician clearance. In consultation with her, you decide that Tanya will exercise three days per week, performing 30 minutes of aerobic work, followed by 30 minutes of flexibility stretching and resistance training, for a total of 60 minutes each session. The first step should be to develop the aerobic workout. You design the program at an intensity that will allow Tanya to exercise continuously for 30 minutes. The advantages of the aerobic program will be to condition the heart, expend calories, and warm up the muscles in preparation for the second phase, which will be the stretches. You decide to have Tanya walk on a treadmill using a target heart rate based on 60 to 80% of her heart rate reserve (HRR). Her estimated maximal HR is 220 − 30 = 190 bpm. You measure her resting HR as 90 bpm.

$$\text{Target HR} = (\text{intensity fraction})(\text{HRmax} - \text{HRrest}) + \text{HRrest}$$

$$\text{Lower target HR} = (0.6)(190 - 90) + 90$$

$$= (0.6)(100) + 90$$

$$= 60 + 90$$

$$= 150 \text{ bpm}$$

$$\text{Upper target HR} = (0.8)(190 - 90) + 90$$

$$= (0.8)(100) + 90$$

$$= 80 + 90$$

$$= 170 \text{ bpm}$$

You instruct Tanya that, once she has completed her aerobic exercise and is thoroughly warmed up, she should perform the static stretches listed in figures 6.1 through 6.5 (in that order), holding each for 15 to 30 seconds, and doing two to four sets of the routine.

In her resistance training program Tanya will use both free weights and machines. Have her start with the upper-body muscles and finish with the lower-body muscles. By following the order in figures 6.6 through 6.14, her first exercises will be compound (those that involve more than one joint, and therefore more than one large muscle or muscle group), and her later exercises will be more isolated (involving only one joint and smaller muscles). To determine the resistance to use, help Tanya pick a weight that she can lift comfortably 8 to 12 times, and increase the weight when she can do 12 repetitions.

CASE STUDY 6.2
Novice Bodybuilder

Carlton is a 24-year-old, 220 lb (100 kg) male who wants to compete in his first bodybuilding contest in five months. Carlton has asked your advice on aerobic and weightlifting exercises. His current body fat percentage is 25%. Carlton feels that he will probably have to be at about 10% body fat to compete in the bodybuilding competition. Although he believes he is in "pretty good shape," you discover that he performs almost no aerobic exercise for fear that he will lose muscle mass. Carlton informs you that he has been lifting weights for five years and believes that his muscle and strength gains have plateaued. Carlton's mother had coronary angioplasty at the age of 53, but he has no other risk factors, signs, or symptoms. He has a resting HR of 85 bpm.

Because Carlton has only one risk factor (family history) and is young (placing him in the low-risk category), you can confidently proceed with his exercise prescription. Given the fact that he has reached a plateau in his training, you prescribe a more advanced routine that involves training specific muscle groups at different times rather than all muscle groups in each workout. Furthermore, because Carlton has been lifting weights and is familiar with the

(continued)

Case Study 6.2   *(continued)*

amount he is able to lift, it is not necessary to calculate a 1RM for each weightlifting exercise. You recommend the following resistance training workout, with each exercise preceded by a warm-up set at a relatively light weight:

- **Frequency:** Twice per week for each routine
- **Duration:** Three sets each of three or four different exercises (totaling 9 to 12 sets) for each body part or muscle group
- **Intensity:** 8 to 10 repetitions per set. When he can perform 10 reps in any one set, increase the weight for that set so that he can perform at least 8 reps. Continue to increase the reps to 10 before adding weight.
- Day 1: Back and biceps exercises
- Day 2: Legs and abdominal muscles
- Day 3: Chest and triceps
- Days 4-6: Repeat days 1-3
- Day 7: Off

Carlton's goal for body composition is to reach 10% fat. This is still fairly high for a competitive bodybuilder, but it is a reasonable goal for his first contest. Determine the amount of fat weight he must lose to accomplish this goal as follows:

$$\text{Goal weight} = (\text{current weight})(1 - \text{current \% fat}) /$$
$$(1 - \text{desired \% fat})$$

$$= (220)(1 - 0.25) / (1 - 0.1)$$

$$= (220)(0.75) / (0.9)$$

$$= 165 / 0.9$$

$$= 183 \text{ lb}$$

Carlton needs to lose 37 lb of fat to reach his goal. Because he has five months to lose this weight, he needs to lose almost 2 lb per week. This gradual weight loss will be important in ensuring that he loses only fat and not muscle. After you reassure Carlton that aerobic exercise, if not done in excess, will not reduce his muscle mass, he agrees to follow your recommendations. For the aerobic portion, because he has 37 lb to lose and because he needs to train his cardiovascular system, you recommend that Carlton do his aerobic exercise at least four times per week. If he does his aerobic workouts on the same days as the resistance training, he should do the resistance training first, because muscular strength and size are his primary goals. You recommend some light stretching before his resistance training, followed by more aggressive stretching after the completion of the aerobic workout.

You decide to use the percent heart rate reserve (%HRR) method for Carlton and prescribe a target heart rate in the range of 60 to 85% HRR. His estimated maximal HR is 220 – 24 = 196 bpm. As reported earlier, his resting HR is 85 bpm.

$$\text{Target HR} = (\text{intensity fraction})(\text{HRmax} - \text{HRrest}) + \text{HRrest}$$

$$\text{Lower target HR} = (0.6)(196 - 85) + 85$$

$$= (0.6)(111) + 85$$

$$= 66.6 + 85$$

$$= 152 \text{ bpm}$$

$$\text{Upper target HR} = (0.85)(196 - 85) + 85$$

$$= (0.85)(111) + 85$$

$$= 94.35 + 85$$

$$= 179 \text{ bpm}$$

Next, because Carlton must lose 37 lb, he wants to know how many calories he is expending during his aerobic exercise so he can adjust his food intake. You can calculate this if you know the $\dot{V}O_2$ during his aerobic exercise. Carlton informs you that to attain his target heart rate, he must jog on the treadmill at 5 mph up an 8% grade. Use the running equation from page 50 to determine his $\dot{V}O_2$. His speed in m · min^{-1} is 5 mph × 26.8 = 134 m · min^{-1}.

$$\dot{V}O_2 = 3.5 + 0.2(\text{speed}) + .9 \text{ (speed)}(\text{fractional grade})$$

$$= 3.5 + 0.2(134) + .9(134)(0.08)$$

$$= 3.5 + 26.8 + 9.6$$

$$= 39.9 \text{ ml · min}^{-1} \cdot \text{kg}^{-1} \text{ (gross } \dot{V}O_2)$$

$$\text{Net } \dot{V}O_2 = 36.4 - 3.5 = 46.1 \text{ ml · min}^{-1} \cdot \text{kg}^{-1}$$

(continued)

Case Study 6.2   *(continued)*

Now that you have calculated Carlton's $\dot{V}O_2$, you can determine the number of calories he burns during a 30-minute aerobic session. Remember to subtract the resting energy expenditure, or 1 MET (3.5 ml · min^{-1} · kg^{-1}), and to report *net* calories burned. To calculate net calories burned, first convert the answer to liters per minute for his entire weight—in this case, 100 kg:

$$\frac{(36.4 \text{ ml} \cdot \text{min}^{-1} \cdot \text{kg}^{-1})(100 \text{ kg})}{1,000} = 3.64 \text{ L} \cdot \text{min}^{-1}$$

Because 5 kcal are expended for each liter of oxygen consumed, during a 30-minute exercise session Carlton would burn the following number of calories:

$$(3.64 \text{ L} \cdot \text{min}^{-1}) \times 5 = 18.2 \text{ kcal} \cdot \text{min}^{-1}$$

$$(18.2 \text{ kcal} \cdot \text{min}^{-1}) \times (30 \text{ min}) = 546 \text{ kcal per a 30-minute}$$
exercise session

Note that 690 kcal are much more than the average person normally burns during 30 minutes of exercise. But Carlton is a large person in fairly good condition. Because he is performing this exercise four times per week, his total caloric expenditure from aerobic exercise is $546 \times 4 = 2{,}184$ kcal per week. This represents $2{,}184 / 3{,}500 = 0.8$ lb of fat. Although his weight training is also greater than it was before, he still needs to adjust his diet to achieve his target of losing nearly 2 lb of fat per week. That is, he should ingest fewer calories each day compared with his diet in the past, especially avoiding fatty foods.

REFERENCES

ACSM. 2006. *ACSM's Guidelines for Exercise Testing and Prescription*, 7th ed., 154-160. Philadelphia: Lippincott Williams & Wilkins.

Baechle, T.R., and R.W. Earle, eds. 2000. *Essentials of Strength Training and Conditioning*, 2nd ed. Champaign, IL: Human Kinetics.

Pollock, M.L., G.A. Gaesser, J.D. Butcher, J.P. Despres, R.K. Dishman, B.A. Franklin, and C.E. Garber. 1998. The recommended quantity and quality of exercise for developing and maintaining cardiorespiratory and muscular fitness, and flexibility in healthy adults (ACSM position stand). *Medicine and Science in Sports and Exercise* 30: 975-991.

7

Exercise Prescription for the Older Adult

Aging is associated with a decline in physical function and, in many cases, a loss of independence. But is aging itself the root cause of these changes? Certainly, some physical decline can be expected as a biological consequence of age, but much of what is called aging is simply the result of years of physical inactivity. Those who remain physically active throughout life demonstrate much slower rates of physical decline than do the sedentary. And a growing body of research indicates that those who have been sedentary for many years can experience significant improvements by beginning an exercise program even at very advanced ages.

As "Adaptations in the Elderly to Exercise Training" on page 102 summarizes, properly prescribed exercise for elderly people can significantly improve their aerobic power (Ehsani, 1987), muscular strength and size (Fiatarone et al., 1990; Fiatarone et al., 1994; Frontera et al., 1988), and bone density (Dalsky, 1989; Menkes et al., 1993). Improvements in functional measures such as walking speed and stair-climbing power have also been reported (Fiatarone et al., 1990; Fiatarone et al., 1994). These results can reverse the effects of many years of physical decline and lead to greater independence and a much higher quality of life.

Adaptations in the Elderly to Exercise Training

- Increased aerobic power ($\dot{V}O_2$max)
- Increased lactate threshold
- Increased muscular strength (1RM)
- Increased muscle cross-sectional area
- Increased bone mineral density
- Increased walking speed
- Increased stair-climbing power

The principles of exercise prescription described in preceding chapters apply to the elderly as well as to younger adults. You may need to modify the guidelines somewhat based on initial fitness level, orthopedic problems, complicating medical conditions, and the effects of medications. Making allowance for these issues *on an individual basis* is the key to adapting the general principles to the elderly.

Do not make the mistake of assuming that all elderly are of a low fitness level. The range of individual variability among the elderly is very large. Whereas some older people are frail and need assistance to accomplish activities of daily living (ADL), others are highly fit and enjoy challenging themselves physically. Many people in their 60s, 70s, and beyond run marathons, participate in century (100-mile) bike rides, do competitive powerlifting, and go on multiday backpacking treks.

The ACSM's *Guidelines* provide specific recommendations for writing exercise prescriptions for the elderly (ACSM, 2006). Although the ACSM offers no special changes from the standard recommendations for flexibility training for the general population, it does prescribe modifications for cardiovascular fitness and resistance training in the elderly.

CARDIOVASCULAR FITNESS

Because many elderly have a low initial fitness level, it is prudent to begin exercise prescriptions at a low intensity and to progress gradually. However, the intensity range of 40 or 50% to 85% of $\dot{V}O_2R$ still applies—just make more frequent use of the low end of this range for initial prescriptions with the elderly. It may even be acceptable to begin at less than 40% on an individual basis.

When prescribing exercise intensity by heart rate, you must consider several factors. Remember that, for adults of any age, formulas for estimating maximal heart rate (such as 220 – age) provide only rough approximations. This is especially true for older adults because the range of actual maximal heart rates grows larger with age. Thus, you should use great caution in applying target HR ranges with elderly clients unless the ranges are based on *measured* maximal heart rates.

Chapter 3 states that the %HRR method is superior to the %HRmax method for establishing target heart rates. Percentage of HRR provides equivalent exercise intensities to %$\dot{V}O_2R$ for older as well as younger adults. A further argument giving preference to the %HRR method is that many elderly have elevated resting heart rates, which causes problems when target heart rates are prescribed by the %HRmax method. As an example in chapter 3 illustrates, the use of %HRmax for elderly clients sometimes results in target heart rates that are little more than people's resting heart rates. *For these reasons, the authors have always recommended %HRR as the preferred method of prescribing target heart rates in the elderly, just as with younger adults.* In the sixth edition of the *Guidelines*, the ACSM indicated a preference for %HRmax when prescribing exercise intensity for the elderly (ACSM, 2000), but the seventh edition of the *Guidelines* recommends the use of %HRR (ACSM, 2006).

The mode of exercise is an important consideration with the elderly, because the best program for counteracting osteoporosis may increase orthopedic problems. To reduce orthopedic stress, you should minimize weight-bearing activities (aquatic exercise is a very good choice). To combat osteoporosis and improve bone density, however, you must maximize weight-bearing activities (which means that aquatic exercise would be a poor choice). The solution to this dilemma is to individualize every program, prescribing weight-bearing exercise *within the client's orthopedic tolerance level.* Walking is an excellent choice for many older people.

Other considerations regarding the mode of exercise include using group exercise as much as possible to engender compliance through social support, and, when choosing aerobic machines, avoiding those with excessively complicated panels and programs.

RESISTANCE TRAINING

The ACSM's recommendations for resistance training for the elderly differ significantly from its standard recommendations for resistance training. As described in this section, and summarized in table 7.1, the present authors take issue with three of these points.

The ACSM specifies that elderly clients should perform 10 to 15 repetitions at a perceived exertion of 12 or 13 ("somewhat hard"), which is in contrast to their recommendation of 8- to 12RM for younger adults. Lifting to the point of failure in 8 to 12 repetitions requires much more effort than performing 10 to 15 repetitions at a level that seems somewhat hard. This is a curious recommendation from the ACSM for two reasons. First, the RPE scale is not generally used for gauging intensity during weightlifting. Second, research with elderly subjects (including nonagenarians) has established that large improvements in strength and modest, yet statistically significant, improvements in muscle size are achieved with sets performed for 8 repetitions at 80% of 1RM (Fiatarone et al., 1990; Fiatarone et al., 1994; Frontera et al., 1988). For most resistance exercises, a weight set at 80% of 1RM can be lifted approximately 10 times. Thus, it would appear that the elderly should use the same 8- to 12-repetition range to failure that is recommended by the ACSM for younger clients. Elderly clients may be using a low absolute intensity (i.e., a low weight) but should not be using a low relative intensity (i.e., % of 1RM).

**Table 7.1 Differences in ACSM's and Authors'
Recommendations for Resistance Training for the Elderly**

Issue	ACSM	Authors
Resistance training intensity	RPE of 12-13	8- to 12RM
Initial adaptation period for resistance training	Eight weeks at minimal resistance	One to two weeks at minimal resistance
Equipment for resistance training	Machines preferred over free weights	Free weights preferred over machines because they stress balance and have smaller weight increments

Clients should choose a weight that they can lift eight times and attempt to perform additional repetitions during succeeding exercise sessions. Once the client is able to lift the weight 12 times, the weight should be increased for the following session. The increase should be small (approximately 10%) and designed to bring the client back to the 8RM level.

Another questionable recommendation by the ACSM is the recommendation that the elderly use minimal resistance for the first eight weeks of a program. The training studies cited earlier used only one week of familiarization before setting the resistance at 80% of 1RM (Fiatarone et al., 1990; Fiatarone et al., 1994; Frontera et al., 1988). One of the authors of this book (Swain) has considerable experience with resistance training with the elderly and uses a one- to two-week period for initial adjustment to the program. This period of time is important for teaching proper lifting technique and for minimizing **delayed-onset muscle soreness (DOMS).** Clients who have not performed resistance exercise for several decades, if ever, must be cautioned to use very light weights on the first day and to still expect DOMS the following day. It is not necessary to attempt 1RM lifts initially, or to find the 8RM by trial and error on the first day of training. Rather, *the weight chosen for the first few sessions should feel easy throughout a set of 12 to 15 repetitions.* The last repetition need not be challenging. Once you are satisfied that the client is using proper form, which should take no longer than two weeks, you can determine the 8RM by trial and error, using that figure to establish the intensity for the progressive phase of training.

A third ACSM recommendation for the elderly that bears some scrutiny is the recommendation to use machines as opposed to free weights. It is true that machines require less skill, but free weights have the advantage of teaching balance and greater neuromuscular control, which may be transferable to real-world activities. Furthermore, free weights are superior for providing small increments of weight. Most exercises can be performed with dumbbells or ankle weights, which come in 1 lb increments at the low end, and 5 lb increments at the high end. A significant disadvantage of machines is that the increments are usually 10 lb or more. A client performing 12 repetitions with 20 lb on a machine is faced with the daunting prospect of moving up to 30 lb, a 50% increase! Fortunately, this can be remedied by attaching a 1 or 2 lb free weight to the machine's weight stack.

The ACSM offers these important recommendations for elderly resistance trainers: Do not exercise during an acute arthritic flare-up; exercise only within a pain-free range of motion; and reduce the load by 50% or more when returning from a layoff. In all other aspects of resistance training, the ACSM's recommendations for the elderly are the same as for younger adults.

CASE STUDY 7.1
Older Adult With Low Initial Fitness

Bart is 82 years old. He is 6'1" (186 cm) tall and weighs 182 lb (82.7 kg). His total cholesterol is 218 mg · dl^{-1}, his LDL is 120 mg · dl^{-1}, his HDL is 43 mg · dl^{-1}, and his fasting glucose is 101 mg · dl^{-1}. He has no family or personal history of heart disease. He has arthritis in his hands and knees, which usually does not prevent him from carrying out activities of daily living. He quit smoking 20 years ago. His blood pressure is 146/86 mmHg, with resting HR of 84 bpm. He plays golf infrequently. He reports no signs or symptoms of cardiopulmonary disease. He has recently undergone a fitness evaluation with the following results: His estimated $\dot{V}O_2$max from a submaximal bike test was 18 ml · min^{-1} · kg^{-1}, he can do three push-ups but no partial (Canadian) curl-ups, and he achieved 23 cm as his sit-and-reach score (on a 26 cm foot-line box). Stratify Bart's risk and assess his fitness. Design a comprehensive exercise prescription for him.

Bart has three risk factors: hypertension, impaired fasting glucose, and a sedentary lifestyle. His BMI is 24 kg · m^{-2}, well below the criterion for risk (which is 30 kg · m^{-2}). His total cholesterol is elevated but is not a risk factor because his LDL is below the threshold of 130 mg · dl^{-1}. His age and his three risk factors place Bart in the moderate-risk category. It would be prudent for him to see his physician concerning his desire to exercise and to discuss the management of his blood glucose, but it is acceptable for him to begin a moderate exercise program at this time. Bart's arthritis is manageable but will need to be considered during his exercise training.

Bart's body composition appears to be normal, although this is based only on BMI. Based on normative tables from chapter 4 of ACSM's seventh edition of the *Guidelines* (ACSM, 2006), his aerobic capacity and muscular strength/endurance are well below average. His sit-and-reach score of 23 cm means that he is not quite able to reach his toes (at the 26 cm mark) and places him at approximately the "good" level. Note, however, that the oldest age range for the ACSM norms is 60 to 69 years, or >65 years (depending on the variable), and may not provide an accurate representation of octogenarians in the population. Appropriate goals for Bart at this time would be to improve his aerobic capacity and muscular strength to the average level for males 60 years old and older, and to maintain or improve his flexibility.

Follow the general guidelines in table 2.1 for Bart's exercise prescription. You begin his cardiovascular conditioning at three sessions per week on alternate days, for 20 minutes per session, at an intensity approximating 40 to 60% of $\dot{V}O_2R$. Given his low initial fitness level, his manageable level of arthritis, and your desire to incorporate weight-bearing activity into his program, you recommend walking as the principal mode of exercise. You should monitor his arthritis symptoms and ask him to back off if they worsen. The simplest way to assign Bart to an intensity of 40 to 60% $\dot{V}O_2R$ may be to use the talk test, or an RPE of 12 to 14 (from table 3.1). Alternatively, you could calculate a target heart rate based on 64 to 77% of HRmax (from table 3.1) or based on 40 to 60% of HRR. These values are 88 to 106 bpm using %HRmax, and 106 to 116 bpm using %HRR (see the following calculations). Given his resting HR of 84 bpm, the values derived from %HRmax would appear to be too low. In either case, because these target HRs were calculated using an estimated HRmax of 220 – age, you understand that they are very rough estimates.

%HRmax method:

$$\text{Lower target HR} = 0.64(220 - 82)$$

$$= 0.64(138)$$

$$= 88 \text{ bpm}$$

$$\text{Upper target HR} = 0.77(138)$$

$$= 106 \text{ bpm}$$

(continued)

Case Study 7.1   *(continued)*

%HRR method:

Target HR = (intensity fraction)(HRmax – HRrest) + HRrest

$$\text{Lower target HR} = 0.40(138 - 84) + 84$$

$$= 0.40(54) + 84$$

$$= 22 + 84$$

$$= 106 \text{ bpm}$$

$$\text{Upper target HR} = 0.60(138 - 84) + 84$$

$$= 0.60(54) + 84$$

$$= 32 + 84$$

$$= 116 \text{ bpm}$$

Another means of setting the intensity would be to calculate a walking speed at 40 to 60% of $\dot{V}O_2R$. Using the walking equation from page 50, this would be 2.2 to 3.2 mph (see the following calculations). This also is only a rough estimate of the exercise intensity, because it is based on an estimated $\dot{V}O_2$max, which furthermore was an estimate made during cycling exercise rather than during walking.

$$\text{Target } \dot{V}O_2 = \text{(intensity fraction)}(\dot{V}O_2\text{max} - 3.5) + 3.5$$

$$\text{Lower target } \dot{V}O_2 = 0.40(18 - 3.5) + 3.5$$

$$= 0.40(14.5) + 3.5$$

$$= 5.8 + 3.5$$

$$= 9.3 \text{ ml} \cdot \text{min}^{-1} \cdot \text{kg}^{-1}$$

$$\text{Upper target } \dot{V}O_2 = 0.60(18 - 3.5) + 3.5$$

$$= 0.60(14.5) + 3.5$$

$$= 8.7 + 3.5$$

$$= 12.2 \text{ ml} \cdot \text{min}^{-1} \cdot \text{kg}^{-1}$$

Now, calculate the desired walking speed using the walking equation from page 50.

$$\dot{V}O_2 = 3.5 + 0.1(\text{speed}) + 1.8(\text{speed})(\text{fractional grade})$$

Lower target workload:

$$9.3 = 3.5 + 0.1(\text{speed}) + 1.8(\text{speed})(0)$$

$$9.3 = 3.5 + 0.1(\text{speed})$$

$$9.3 - 3.5 = 0.1(\text{speed})$$

$$5.8 = 0.1(\text{speed})$$

$$5.8 / 0.1 = \text{speed}$$

$$58 \text{ m} \cdot \text{min}^{-1} = \text{speed}$$

$$(58 \text{ m} \cdot \text{min}^{-1}) / 26.8 = 2.2 \text{ mph}$$

Upper target workload:

$$12.2 = 3.5 + 0.1(\text{speed})$$

$$12.2 - 3.5 = 0.1(\text{speed})$$

$$8.7 = 0.1(\text{speed})$$

$$8.7 / 0.1 = \text{speed}$$

$$87 \text{ m} \cdot \text{min}^{-1} = \text{speed}$$

$$(87 \text{ m} \cdot \text{min}^{-1}) / 26.8 = 3.2 \text{ mph}$$

To summarize, you can estimate the intensity as a HR or walking speed, but you must closely observe Bart's responses to the exercise to determine whether he appears to be exercising at a light to moderate level. If he has difficulty completing 20 minutes at this level, you need to reduce the intensity. (Alternatively, he could perform two 10-minute bouts with a rest period in between.) If he finds that 20 minutes at this level is very easy, increase the intensity until it reaches a moderate level (termed "somewhat hard" on the Borg scale). Once you have established the proper intensity, Bart can enter the improvement phase, in which he gradually increases the duration and frequency of his cardiovascular exercise. Furthermore, as his ability improves, he can increase his absolute intensity (i.e., walking speed) while leaving his relative intensity (i.e., HR) within the target range.

(continued)

Case Study 7.1   *(continued)*

Bart should perform his resistance training program two or three times per week. If he is exercising in your facility three times per week for cardiovascular conditioning, it might be useful to have him perform his resistance training as part of the same sessions. Teach him how to properly perform a variety of exercises that target all of the major muscle groups. Pay special attention to lifting technique, range of motion through a pain-free arc, proper breathing (avoiding the Valsalva maneuver), and a controlled speed of movement through both the concentric (lifting) and eccentric (lowering) phases. He should begin with very light weights while learning proper technique. Once he has developed skill at the various lifts and has overcome his initial soreness, help Bart select weights that provide the appropriate intensity for the improvement phase of the program (10 to 15 "somewhat hard" repetitions in accordance with ACSM guidelines, or 8 to 12 repetitions to volitional fatigue if you follow the authors' recommendations). He should perform at least one set of each of the selected exercises. A preferred routine might be to perform one set at 50% of the prescribed intensity as a warm-up, and then one or two sets at the prescribed intensity. The routine should allow completion of all lifts in no more than one hour, and preferably in 20 to 30 minutes.

Bart does not need to place a lot of emphasis on the flexibility aspect of his training program, at least with regard to his measured lower-back and hamstring flexibility. However, to ensure maintenance of good all-round flexibility, at the conclusion of each exercise session he should perform a variety of flexibility exercises targeting all major muscle groups. These exercises should follow the general guidelines summarized in table 2.1, in which each stretch is taken to a point of tightness and held for 15 to 30 seconds. He should perform each stretch two to four times.

CASE STUDY 7.2
Older Adult With High Initial Fitness

Francine is 66 years old. She is 5'5" tall and weighs 136 lb. A long-distance cyclist who has ridden across several states, she averages 10 to 15 hours of bicycling per week. Her total cholesterol is 193 mg · dl^{-1}, her LDL is 102 mg · dl^{-1}, her HDL is 64 mg · dl^{-1}, and her fasting glucose is 88 mg · dl^{-1}. Her father had a heart attack at 53 years of age. She is a nonsmoker. Her blood pressure is 118/74 mmHg, and her resting HR is 62 bpm. She reports no signs or symptoms of cardiopulmonary disease. A recent fitness evaluation yielded the following results: 44 ml $\cdot$ min^{-1} $\cdot$ kg^{-1} estimated $\dot{V}O_2$max from a submaximal bike test, 45 lb for a 1RM bench press, 170 lb for a 1RM leg press, 10 modified push-ups, three partial (Canadian) curl-ups, and a 21 cm sit-and-reach score (on a 26 cm foot-line box). Stratify Francine's risk and assess her fitness. Design a comprehensive exercise prescription for her.

Francine has only one risk factor: family history. However, because she has the negative risk factor of a high HDL level (above 60 mg $\cdot$ dl^{-1}), we would count her as having zero risk factors for screening purposes. Nevertheless, Francine is in the moderate-risk category because of her age. You can safely place her in a moderate-intensity exercise program.

Francine's body composition is considered normal, based on a BMI of 22.6 kg $\cdot$ m^{-2}. Her aerobic capacity of 44 ml $\cdot$ min^{-1} $\cdot$ kg^{-1} is excellent for her age group, being in the 90th percentile based on the table of norms in chapter 4 of the seventh edition of the ACSM's *Guidelines* (ACSM, 2006). Her muscular fitness presents a mixed picture. You can evaluate her upper-body strength from her bench press 1RM, expressed as a fraction of her body weight (45 / 136 = 0.33). This value places her in the 10th percentile. Her lower-body strength is much better: Her 1RM/body weight ratio for the leg press is 1.25, placing her at approximately the 85th percentile. Her upper-body muscular endurance is better than her upper-body strength, because her 10 modified push-ups place her approximately at the "good" level. Her abdominal muscle endurance is not as good, with three partial curl-ups placing her at the low end of the "fair" range. Finally, the flexibility of her lower back and hamstrings, as indicated by a sit-and-reach score of 21 cm, places her in the "needs improvement" category. In summary, although Francine has very good aerobic capacity and leg strength from her bicycling, she needs to improve in other areas. Goals for Francine would be to maintain her aerobic capacity and leg strength, and to improve to at least the average level her muscular strength, muscular endurance, and flexibility.

Francine does not need any guidance regarding her cardiovascular conditioning. If she wants a target range, you could suggest

(continued)

Case Study 7.2 *(continued)*

60 to 80% of $\dot{V}O_2R$. From table 3.1, you could estimate this intensity as 77 to 91% of HRmax, or 119 to 140 bpm; or, using 60 to 80% of HRR, her target HRs would be 117 to 136 bpm (see the following calculations). Note that, because she has a low resting HR, the %HRmax and %HRR methods yield similar answers. However, you should use caution in applying these values, because they were calculated with HRmax estimated as 220 – age.

%HRmax method:

$$\text{Lower target HR} = 0.77(220 - 66)$$

$$= 0.77(154)$$

$$= 119 \text{ bpm}$$

$$\text{Upper target HR} = 0.91(154)$$

$$= 140 \text{ bpm}$$

%HRR method:

$$\text{Target HR} = (\text{intensity fraction})(\text{HRmax} - \text{HRrest}) + \text{HRrest}$$

$$\text{Lower target HR} = 0.60(154 - 62) + 62$$

$$= 0.60(92) + 62$$

$$= 55 + 62$$

$$= 117 \text{ bpm}$$

$$\text{Upper target HR} = 0.80(154 - 62) + 62$$

$$= 0.80(92) + 62$$

$$= 74 + 62$$

$$= 136 \text{ bpm}$$

Francine would definitely benefit from a resistance training program. Given her excellent leg strength, she should emphasize upper-body and trunk exercises. However, she also should include leg exercises to balance her development. Like Bart, discussed earlier, she should perform her resistance training program two or three days per week, using at least one set of each exercise performed at a "somewhat hard" level for 10 to 15 repetitions (to follow ACSM guidelines), or at an 8- to 12RM load (to follow the recommendations of the authors).

Francine should follow a well-designed flexibility program that includes a variety of stretches that target all major muscle groups (with special attention to her lower-back and hamstring area, which needs improvement) and that are performed for two to four repetitions of 15 to 30 seconds, each to a point of tightness. Rather than limiting herself to doing these exercises after her resistance training two or three times per week, she also should stretch after her aerobic workouts, which she does on an almost daily basis.

REFERENCES

ACSM. 2000. *ACSM's Guidelines for Exercise Testing and Prescription*, 6th ed., 223-230. Philadelphia: Lippincott Williams & Wilkins.

ACSM, 2006. *ACSM's Guidelines for Exercise Testing and Prescription*, 7th ed., 79-89, 246-250. Philadelphia: Lippincott Williams & Wilkins.

Dalsky, G.P. 1989. The role of exercise in the prevention of osteoporosis. *Comprehensive Therapy* 15 (9): 30-37.

Ehsani, A.A. 1987. Cardiovascular adaptations to exercise training in the elderly. *Federation Proceedings* 46: 1840-1843.

Fiatarone, M.A., E.C. Marks, N.D. Ryan, C.N. Meredith, L.A. Lipsitz, and W.J. Evans. 1990. High intensity strength training in nonagenarians. *Journal of the American Medical Association* 263: 3029-3034.

Fiatarone, M.A., E.F. O'Neill, N.D. Ryan, K.M. Clements, G.R. Solares, M.E. Nelson, S.B. Roberts, J.J. Kehayias, L.A. Lipsitz, and W.J. Evans. 1994. Exercise training and nutritional supplementation for physical frailty in very elderly people. *New England Journal of Medicine* 330: 1769-1775.

Frontera, W.R., C.N. Meredith, K.P. O'Reilly, H.G. Knuttgen, and W.J. Evans. 1988. Strength conditioning in older men: Skeletal muscle hypertrophy and improved function. *Journal of Applied Physiology* 64: 1038-1044.

Menkes A., S. Mazel, R.A. Redmond, K. Koffler, C.R. Libinati, C.M. Gundberg, T.M. Zizic, J.M. Hagberg, R.E. Pratley, and B.F. Hurley. 1993. Strength training increases regional bone mineral density and bone remodeling in middle-aged and older men. *Journal of Applied Physiology* 74: 2478-2484.

8

Exercise Prescription
for Heart Disease

Heart disease, or **coronary artery disease,** is the number one cause of death in the United States. When a person exercises, the heart must work harder, and its demand for blood flow and oxygen increases. A person with clinically significant coronary artery disease cannot increase the flow of blood and oxygen to the heart sufficiently during such times of increased demand, which can result in chest pain, or **angina.** Angina may result when a coronary artery is blocked 50% or more, as seen on an angiographic view of the artery during a heart catheterization (Wenger and Hellerstein, 1992). It is important to realize that a 50% reduction in lumen diameter translates to a 75% reduction in the cross-sectional area of the lumen (the opening in an artery through which blood flows). Moreover, angiography typically underestimates the true extent of blockage, because the narrowed section of artery is being compared to adjacent sections, and these adjacent sections are likely also narrowed as a result of the diffuse presence of plaque throughout the diseased artery. Most people do not notice heart disease resulting from atherosclerosis, or blocked arteries, until they experience significant symptoms or damage. Other types of heart disease may result from valve damage and high blood pressure. **Myocardial infarctions (MIs)** can cause extensive damage to the heart that can result in congestive heart failure. Some patients may even require pacemakers or automated defibrillators for the management of **arrhythmias.**

EXERCISE FOR HEART DISEASE

Exercise benefits people with heart disease in many ways. Regular exercise decreases sympathetic drive, which reduces both blood pressure and heart rate during submaximal exercise and at rest. This means that the patient can perform a given amount of work with less demand (a lower rate–pressure product) on the heart. Reduced sympathetic drive also decreases ventricular irritability, which can diminish the risk of serious arrhythmias.

Regular exercise also reduces the risk for further progression of heart disease by reducing LDL cholesterol, increasing HDL cholesterol, reducing obesity, and reducing sympathetically mediated blood pressure and platelet stickiness. One study that incorporated regular exercise with a low-fat diet and stress reduction found that such a comprehensive plan resulted in actual regression of coronary blockage (Ornish et al., 1990). In that study, the subjects who performed the most exercise, averaging an hour a day at a moderate intensity, achieved the best results. Other benefits of exercise for heart disease patients include a reduction in health care costs, a faster return to daily activities after hospitalization, and improvements in functional capacity and self-esteem.

FOUR VARIABLES OF THE FITT PRINCIPLE

Aerobic exercise prescriptions for patients with heart disease should include the four basic variables of the FITT principle: frequency, intensity, time (duration), and type (mode). Weightlifting also may be added once a regular program of aerobic exercise has been established. You must modify the basic guidelines for exercise prescription according to the client's clinical status and the phase of rehabilitation.

Standard cardiac rehabilitation programs have four phases. Phase I (inpatient) is usually short (three to five days) and involves patient care in the hospital under the direct supervision of a physician and either a nurse, exercise specialist, or physical therapist. Phase II (outpatient) follows hospital discharge and requires the patient to return to the hospital for rehabilitation, usually lasting 12 weeks. However, many phase II programs now stratify patients according to risk status. Some insurance carriers provide only limited coverage for lower risk patients, and therefore low-, moderate-, and high-risk patients may train for 6, 8, or 12 weeks, respectively. This phase includes ECG and blood pressure monitoring for most patients, and education. Phase III (community-initial) and phase IV (community-maintenance) are usually held at a university, health club, or other fitness setting. They are variable in length and include little supervision and monitoring. To be admitted to phase III or IV programs, patients must be clinically stable, must have normal blood pressure and ECG responses to exercise, and should have a functional capacity of least 8 METs. Patients engaging in inpatient, outpatient, or community exercise should be risk stratified according to medical history, clinical status, and symptoms.

The exercise prescription during phase I depends strongly on the clinical status of the patient. According to the FITT principle, here is a general exercise prescription for most inpatients:

- **Frequency:** Some type of mobilization at least twice a day (three or four times per day initially) to prevent stasis and clotting of blood.
- **Intensity:** An RPE less than 13, or target heart rate that is 20 bpm above the standing resting HR for post-MI patients (not to exceed 120 bpm), or 30 bpm above standing resting HR for postsurgery patients.
- **Time:** Intermittent bouts lasting 3 to 5 minutes, with rest periods shorter than the mobilization time (as tolerated by the patient), for a total time of 20 minutes.
- **Type:** Mobilization activities such as sitting up in bed with or without assistance, self-care activities, walking in the halls of the hospital, or stationary cycle activity.

Exercise prescription for patients involved in phases II through IV are also contingent on clinical status, but emphasize education and activities designed to help them return to their premorbid lifestyle. A general exercise prescription for most outpatients that follows the FITT principle is as follows:

- **Frequency:** A minimum of two days per week appears to be effective for cardiorespiratory conditioning.
- **Intensity:** The minimum effective intensity of training for cardiac patients is approximately 45% of oxygen uptake reserve ($\dot{V}O_2R$) (Swain and Franklin, 2002). Thus, 45 to 85% $\dot{V}O_2R$ is the

full range that may be considered, which can be translated into a target heart rate or workload as described in chapter 3; most prescriptions focus on the lower end of this range, depending on patient status. With many patients, the intensity will be based on signs or symptoms of ischemia: for example, using a target heart rate that is 10 bpm below the onset of ST-segment depression or the onset of angina, as established during a stress test (ACSM, 2006). A depression of the ST-segment on the ECG of at least 1 mm during exercise suggests coronary ischemia. Such ischemia may be associated with angina but may also occur without any symptoms (termed "silent" ischemia).

- **Time:** To achieve a training effect, 20 to 60 minutes of continuous or intermittent exercise is required. Patients should progress toward a minimum goal of 1,000 kcal per week over a three- to six-month period.

- **Type:** Both aerobic and resistance training are used. A variety of equipment is recommended—treadmills, cycle and arm ergometers, steppers, rowers, and weight machines. Phases III and IV may include skilled games such as basketball and volleyball.

Many cardiac patients are very deconditioned either pre- or postsurgery (or both), or when they enter or complete a cardiac rehabilitation program. It is not unusual for patients entering and leaving cardiac rehab programs to have a 3 and 5 MET capacity, respectively. To help strengthen and improve self-confidence, resistance training may be prescribed, most often during outpatient rehabilitation. Resistance training appears to reduce cardiac demands during daily activities by lowering the rate–pressure product, or myocardial oxygen consumption (ACSM, 2006). Eligibility for resistance training programs is most often decided by the medical director or clinical exercise physiologist. This decision is based on the following guidelines:

- Five weeks following cardiac MI or surgery, including four weeks of supervised rehabilitation

- Three weeks following angioplasty (i.e., percutaneous transluminal coronary angioplasty [PTCA] with or without placement of a stent), including two weeks of supervised rehabilitation

- No current evidence of congestive heart failure, uncontrolled arrhythmias or hyptertension, severe valve disease, or unstable symptoms

Most resistance training programs for cardiac patients include using low weight (e.g., 40 to 50% of the maximal voluntary contraction [1RM] and high [10-15] repetitions in a circuit type program that involves one set for each machine or body part). Additionally, patients should be instructed on proper lifting techniques and avoid the Vasalva maneuver to control blood pressure and the rate–pressure product. Perceived exertions should range from 11 to 13 ("light" to "somewhat hard" on the Borg scale).

MYOCARDIAL INFARCTION

A few decades ago, people who experienced a heart attack were placed on bed rest for several weeks. Today it is well recognized that bed rest worsens the patient's condition and that early mobilization followed by exercise training is an important means of restoring activities of daily living, improving fitness, and reducing risk factors for the further progression of the disease. People who have experienced an MI typically report severe chest pressure or pain that radiates to the left arm, back, or neck. This is usually accompanied by nausea and diaphoresis (sweating). Upon admission to an emergency room, patients are observed to have ECG changes, usually ST elevation, high levels of cardiac enzymes (e.g., CK-MB bands), and chest pain that is relieved by nitroglycerin.

Two types of myocardial infarctions are generally described and progress from the inner muscle of the heart, where pressures and tensions are greatest, outward to the epicardium or outer surface. The first is a **transmural infarction**, which involves the entire thickness of the heart muscle and is represented by a deep or diagnostic Q wave on the ECG. The second type is a **subendocardial infarction** or "non Q wave infarction." It is limited to the inner half of the myocardium. Many times a subendocardial infarction will progress to a transmural infarction if ignored. The three arteries most often blocked by an MI are the left anterior descending (or left coronary artery), the circumflex, and the right coronary artery (Durstine and Moore, 2003).

Myocardial Infarction Patient

A 44-year-old, 179 lb corporate executive, Samir, was admitted to the hospital complaining of chest pain. After evaluating Samir, the cardiologist determined that he was experiencing a mild heart attack, or MI. He was immediately taken to the catheterization lab, where he was diagnosed with a significantly blocked left circumflex artery. A PTCA was performed. A follow-up echocardiography test reported an ejection fraction of 55%, indicating that Samir had not suffered major heart damage. Two weeks later, Samir was referred to you for an exercise prescription in a phase II cardiac rehabilitation program. His only medication is daily aspirin. A maximal treadmill exercise test taking Samir to volitional fatigue after his PTCA revealed the following information:

- **ECG:** Normal sinus rhythm
- **Maximal heart rate:** 156 bpm
- **Resting heart rate:** 62 bpm
- **Peak blood pressure:** 150/90 mmHg
- **Resting blood pressure:** 120/70 mmHg

Because Samir's heart did not sustain a large amount of damage, and because of his younger age and desire to exercise, you choose a fairly moderate to vigorous window for his intensity, such as 60 to 80% of $\dot{V}O_2R$ using the %HRR method. He will work up to 45 minutes of this exercise during his phase II sessions, which will be held three times per week.

$$\text{Target HR} = (\text{intensity fraction})(\text{HRmax} - \text{HRrest}) + \text{HRrest}$$

$$\text{Lower target HR} = (0.60)(156 - 62) + 62$$

$$= (0.60)(94) + 62$$

$$= 56 + 62$$

$$= 118 \text{ bpm}$$

$$\text{Upper target HR} = (0.80)(156 - 62) + 62$$

$$= (0.80)(94) + 62$$

$$= 75 + 62$$

$$= 137 \text{ bpm}$$

If Samir performs the exercise as prescribed, will he reach the goal of expending at least 1,000 kcal per week? Samir tells you that to exercise in his target heart rate range, he must jog on a treadmill at 4 mph, 3% grade. To calculate the $\dot{V}O_2$ for Samir, use the running equation from page 50. His running speed in m·min^{-1} is 4 mph $\times$ 26.8 = 107.2 m·min^{-1}.

$$\dot{V}O_2 = 3.5 + 0.2(\text{speed}) + 0.9(\text{speed})(\text{fractional grade})$$
$$= 3.5 + 0.2(107.2) + 0.9(107.2)(0.03)$$
$$= 3.5 + 21.4 + 2.9$$
$$= 27.8 \text{ ml·min}^{-1}\text{·kg}^{-1} \text{ (gross } \dot{V}O_2)$$

Net $\dot{V}O_2 = 27.8 - 3.5 = 24.3$ ml·min^{-1}·kg^{-1}

To calculate *net* calories burned, first convert the answer to liters per minute. Samir's body mass is (179 lb) / 2.2 = 81.4 kg.

$$\frac{(24.3 \text{ ml·min}^{-1}\text{·kg}^{-1})(81.4 \text{ kg})}{1,000} = 1.98 \text{ L·min}^{-1}$$

Because 5 kcal are expended for each liter of oxygen consumed, Samir would burn the following number of calories:

$$(1.98 \text{ L·min}^{-1}) \times 5 = 9.9 \text{ kcal·min}^{-1}$$
$$(9.9 \text{ kcal·min}^{-1}) \times (45 \text{ min})$$
$$= 445 \text{ kcal per exercise session}$$

Phase II meets three times per week, so Samir would burn 445 $\times$ 3 = 1,338 kcal, exceeding the minimum recommended weekly caloric expenditure.

CONGESTIVE HEART FAILURE

People who suffer significant left ventricular damage after a myocardial infarction will have diminished cardiac output that may progressively worsen and result in peripheral and pulmonary edema. These patients characteristically have a depressed systolic function, diastolic function, or both. Symptoms typically include water retention, weight gain, orthopnea (difficulty in breathing when lying down), and fatigue. It is not uncommon for patients with severe **congestive heart failure (CHF)** to eventually receive cardiac transplants. Ejection fractions less than 50% at rest indicate a moderate risk, whereas ejection fractions less than 40% indicate a high risk of developing CHF. Nonetheless, people with CHF respond positively to an exercise training program, which can improve functional capacity, reduce symptoms, and improve quality of life. However, ejection fractions have not been reported to significantly improve following exercise programs in the majority of studies. Patients who have CHF and are selected for exercise must be stable and should have an exercise capacity of at least 3 METs. Because many of these patients will be taking a myriad of medications (e.g., ACE inhibitors, beta-blockers, diuretics, and antiarrhythmics), a thorough understanding of these medications and how they affect exercise is essential for the exercise physiologist.

CASE STUDY 8.2
Congestive Heart Failure Patient

Phillip is a 65-year-old retired salesman with a 20-year history of heart disease that includes two myocardial infarctions, each followed by a bypass operation. The most recent bypass was last year. He has decided to begin an exercise program, but because he is experiencing shortness of breath, Phillip has wisely decided to seek the recommendation of his physician. The physician ordered a cardiopulmonary exercise stress test and an echocardiography test to evaluate Phillip's heart and exercise capacity. The exercise stress test was performed on a treadmill using the modified Bruce protocol and was terminated at volitional exhaustion. Although Phillip reported no cardiac symptoms during the exercise stress test, he had to end the test after just five minutes because of shortness of breath. His echocardiography test reported a low ejection fraction, about 30%. His physician determined that Phillip was in congestive heart failure, and he prescribed a diuretic, an ACE inhibitor, and a K^+ supplement. His physician cleared Phillip for exercise and referred him to you. The results of the cardiopulmonary exercise stress test were as follows:

- **ECG:** Old myocardial infarctions (significant Q wave present)
- **Maximal heart rate:** 115 beats per minute (test stopped as a result of dyspnea)

- **Resting heart rate:** 85 bpm
- **Peak blood pressure:** 150/90 mmHg
- **Resting blood pressure:** 100/80 mmHg
- **V̇O₂max:** 12 ml · min⁻¹ · kg⁻¹

After meeting with Phillip, you decide to prescribe a low-intensity exercise program using the FITT principle and following ACSM guidelines.

Frequency: Many patients with chronic CHF such as Phillip become very tired after exercise. Exercise sessions of three to seven days per week are recommended.

Intensity: A target heart rate corresponding to 40 to 75% of V̇O₂max or an RPE of 11 to 14 is standard. Note that the ACSM has changed the basis for cardiorespiratory exercise prescription from %V̇O₂max to %V̇O₂R for most situations; however, it retains the terminology of %V̇O₂max for certain special populations (ACSM, 2006). Because Phillip performed very poorly on his modified Bruce treadmill test, and dyspnea was the limiting factor, you prescribe exercise based on an RPE of 11 to 14 rather than determining a target HR. Phillip will need to tailor his intensity according to his dyspnea (for more information on dyspnea, see case study 10.2).

Time: After a prolonged warm-up period of 10 to 15 minutes, exercise intervals as brief as 2 to 6 minutes may be required. Initially you set a goal of 10 to 20 minutes for Phillip, with instructions to progressively lengthen this period to 40 minutes.

Type: You prescribe walking, stationary cycling, and other aerobic activities that Phillip can tolerate well. Later, Phillip can add resistance training using high repetitions and low weight, not more frequently than three days per week.

PACEMAKERS

Exercise recommendations for people with pacemakers vary according to the type of pacemaker. The first type of pacemaker—represented by the acronym VVI—is used to manage **ventricular bradycardias.** The disadvantage of this device is that it does not allow the heart rate, and therefore cardiac output, to increase normally during exercise. The pacemaker is set at a fixed heart rate, so exercise prescriptions using target heart rates are inappropriate. For these patients, exercise intensity should be prescribed by perceived exertion or MET level. Exercise blood pressure also may be used to monitor and prescribe exercise intensity. The Karvonen equation can be used by substituting systolic blood pressure for heart rate. A fractional percentage of 0.50 to 0.80 can be used to calculate a training systolic blood pressure. However, using this method requires that the maximum systolic blood pressure be measured during an incremental exercise test. For a complete description of pacemakers and their codes, see the seventh edition of the ACSM *Guidelines*.

The second type of pacemaker is **rate-responsive** and rate-modulated, allowing heart rate and cardiac output to increase with exercise. This type of pacemaker—the acronym is DDD, DDDR, or VVIR—most closely mimics the heart's normal control. For these patients, exercise can be prescribed using a target heart rate, as well as by workload based on $\dot{V}O_2$ or RPE. The intensity should be approximate 50 to 85% of the HRR, four to seven days per week, for 20 to 60 minutes each session.

The final type of pacemaker is an **antitachycardic** pacemaker, or ICD. These pacemakers manage rapid heart rates by delivering an electric shock to the heart. You can use standard ACSM guidelines to prescribe exercise for these patients—just be certain that you know the upper limits of the ICD, so you won't prescribe a heart rate that will elicit inappropriate shocks during exercise! Typically, heart rates are set 10 to 20 beats below the "cutoff" point to prevent any chance of unnecessary shocks during exercise.

In most cases, resistance training or any upper-body activity that involves the hands being lifted over the shoulders should be avoided for at least two weeks following any type of pacemaker implantation.

CASE STUDY 8.3
Patient With Pacemaker

Cecelia has recently had a VVI pacemaker installed to manage ventricular bradycardia. Cecelia had been feeling very tired, which brought this condition to the attention of a physician. As a result of the nature of Cecelia's pacemaker, her heart rate is set at a fixed rate of 120 beats per minute. Her resting and peak blood pressures are 100/80 and 140/84 mmHg, respectively. She has been referred to your phase III and IV outpatient cardiac rehabilitation program for exercise.

Following ACSM guidelines, you develop the following exercise prescription for Cecelia, according to the FITT principle:

Frequency: You recommend four to seven days per week and encourage her to be active on days outside of her rehabilitation session.

Intensity: An intensity of 50 to 85% of HRR can be used for patients with rate-responsive pacemakers. But Cecelia has a fixed-rate pacemaker and will not demonstrate a linear relationship between heart rate and oxygen consumption. Prescribing exercise by target heart rate is not appropriate. You can prescribe intensity according to RPE, a target workload based on $\dot{V}O_2$, or a modified Karvonen formula for blood pressure. The modified Karvonen formula substitutes **systolic blood pressure (SBP)** for heart rate. The following is a calculation of a target systolic blood pressure for Cecelia at intensities of 50% and 85%, using a modified Karvonen formula:

$$Target\ SBP = (intensity\ fraction)(SBPmax - SBPrest) + SBPrest$$

$$Lower\ target\ SBP = (0.50)(140 - 100) + 100$$

$$= (0.50)(40) + 100$$

$$= 20 + 100$$

$$= 120\ mmHg$$

$$Upper\ target\ SBP = (0.85)(140 - 100) + 100$$

$$= (0.85)(40) + 100$$

$$= 34 + 100$$

$$= 134\ mmHg$$

Time: Most phase III and IV cardiac rehabilitation programs consist of 60-minute time slots for exercise. You prescribe interval training at first, followed by progressive increases in exercise time to achieve 20 to 60 minutes per session.

(continued)

Case Study 8.3   *(continued)*

Type: You prescribe walking, cycling, swimming, and other aerobic activities that involve large muscle groups. Low- to moderate-intensity resistance training may be indicated but should not begin until two or three weeks after implantation of the pacemaker to avoid dislodging implanted leads.

CARDIAC TRANSPLANT

People with severe, untreatable cardiac disease, such as advanced congestive heart failure, may be eligible for cardiac transplantation. Donor hearts are in very short supply. However, as many as 3,000 patients in end-stage heart failure are eligible for a transplant each year. Unfortunately, there is only a three-year survival rate for these patients. It is not unusual for these patients to suffer from dyslipidemias, hypertension, obesity, and diabetes, and be very inactive, which places their donor heart at risk for coronary atherosclerosis. Typical medications include cyclosporin and prednisone to prevent rejection. Hypertension is commonly associated with cyclosporin, and prednisone has numerous side effects such as diabetes, fluid retention, loss of muscle mass, osteoporosis, increased appetite, and other metabolic conditions.

Transplant recipients present a unique situation to the exercise professional. Of special concern are the physiological responses of the denervated heart, as well as the possibility of tissue rejection. As a result of the denervation, two separate P waves may be present on the ECG. Patients often demonstrate resting tachycardia, which may result from circulating norepinephrine and lack of parasympathetic control, and little if any increase in heart rate when exercising. Cardiac output increases are seen as a result of augmented catecholamine levels (stroke volume) and increases in preload, which results when the working muscles help to deliver blood to the heart during activity (Frank-Starling mechanism). Because cardiac transplant patients have about a 50% reduction in maximal oxygen capacity, when exercising they often experience an early onset of anaerobiosis. Longer warm-ups and cool-downs are recommended prior to exercise to account for slower physiological responses to exercise.

CASE STUDY 8.4
Cardiac Transplant Patient

Phillip, the 65-year-old retired salesman described in case study 8.2 with a history of congestive heart failure, became a candidate for a cardiac transplant because his condition had progressed to end-stage heart failure. After his transplant, Phillip was referred to your phase II cardiac rehabilitation program for exercise.

Using the FITT principle, and following ACSM guidelines, you devise the following exercise prescription:

Frequency: Phillip should do aerobic exercise four to six days per week. (Encourage people enrolled in rehabilitation programs that meet only three days per week to exercise on off days. They can perform range-of-motion and resistance training two or three days per week.)

Intensity: Because transplantation surgery denervates the heart, heart rate does not increase during exercise (other than a small increase over time as a result of circulating catecholamines). You therefore cannot prescribe exercise by heart rate. The ACSM recommends that you set exercise intensity at a target workload based on 50 to 75% peak $\dot{V}O_2$ or an RPE of 11 to 15 (ACSM, 2006). If cardiopulmonary data are available, you can base the intensity on the ventilatory threshold. In some cases, you may need to use the dyspnea scale (see case study 10.2). Phillip was unable to perform a maximal cardiorespiratory exercise test because of early exhaustion, so you can base his exercise intensity on the RPE scale using a range of 11 to 15.

Time: You indicate that Phillip should begin his sessions with at least 15 minutes of continuous exercise, progressing to 60 minutes.

Type: Any aerobic exercise that works large muscle groups is appropriate (e.g., walking, jogging, cycling, swimming, stepping, and rowing). You also encourage Phillip to engage in resistance training to prevent glucocorticoid-induced myopathy and losses of lean body mass.

During Phillip's exercise, you should focus on recognizing the adverse effects of immunosuppressive drug therapy and on

(continued)

recognizing the possibility of rejection. *Some important possible consequences of immunosuppressive therapy include hypertension, loss of muscle mass, glucose intolerance, and osteoporosis.* If you note any sign of rejection, Phillip should discontinue his exercise until the rejection is reversed.

REFERENCES

ACSM. 2006. *ACSM's Guidelines for Exercise Testing and Prescription,* 7th ed., 174-201. Philadelphia: Lippincott Williams & Wilkins.

Durstine, J.L., and G.E Moore. 2003. *ACSM's Exercise Management for Persons With Chronic Diseases and Disabilities,* 2nd ed. Champaign, IL: Human Kinetics.

Ornish, D., S.E. Brown, L.W. Scherwitz, J.H. Billings, W.T. Armstrong, T.A. Ports, and S.M. McLanahan. 1990. Can lifestyle changes reverse coronary heart disease? The Lifestyle Heart Trial. *Lancet* 336: 129-133.

Swain, D.P., and B.A. Franklin. 2002. Is there a threshold intensity for aerobic training in cardiac patients? *Medicine and Science in Sports and Exercise* 34: 1071-1075.

Wenger, K.N., and H.K. Hellerstein. 1992. *Rehabilitation of the Coronary Patient,* 3rd ed., 25-26. New York: Churchill Livingstone.

9

Exercise Prescription for Diabetes Mellitus

Exercise prescription for a client with diabetes depends on the type of diabetes the client has. There are two principal types of diabetes mellitus. In type 1 diabetes, a relatively rare disorder that usually begins in childhood, the person's immune system destroys the insulin-producing cells of the pancreas. As a result, glucose cannot enter most cells in the body and builds up in the bloodstream. The person must inject insulin regularly for survival. Type 1 diabetes was formerly known as juvenile-onset diabetes, or insulin-dependent diabetes mellitus (IDDM).

Type 2 diabetes is much more common than type 1, accounting for over 90% of all cases of diabetes. In type 2 diabetes, cells throughout the body become less sensitive to insulin. Insulin is still made by the pancreas, but it is progressively less effective at moving glucose into the cells. This loss of insulin sensitivity is strongly related to both inactivity and obesity. Type 2 diabetes was once found almost exclusively in middle-aged or older adults, but with the growing obesity epidemic it is becoming increasingly more common in children. Type 2 diabetes was formerly known as adult-onset diabetes, or as non-insulin-dependent diabetes mellitus (NIDDM). The latter term was especially misleading because many type 2 patients "progress" in their treatment from (1) exercise and diet, to (2) oral drugs that either stimulate insulin secretion or increase tissue sensitivity to insulin, to (3) insulin injections. Thus, some type 2 patients are in fact dependent on exogenous insulin.

Other categories of diabetes mellitus that are closely related to type 2 are impaired fasting glucose (IFG), impaired glucose tolerance (IGT), and gestational diabetes mellitus (GDM). IFG and IGT are related terms that signify the early stage of type 2 diabetes, before a person reaches the criteria for a diagnosis of diabetes. Diabetes is usually diagnosed as fasting blood glucose levels ≥ 126 mg $\cdot$ dl^{-1}, but it can also be diagnosed from symptoms and random blood glucose values or from the results of a glucose tolerance test (Expert Committee, 2003). **Impaired fasting glucose** is defined as fasting blood glucose levels from 100 to 125 mg $\cdot$ dl^{-1} (note that the threshold was lowered from 110 to 100 mg $\cdot$ dl^{-1} in 2003). **Impaired glucose tolerance** is basically the same condition as IFG but is based on the results of a glucose tolerance test rather than on fasting blood glucose. For a glucose tolerance test, the person drinks a glucose solution, and blood glucose is measured over the next three hours to observe how high it rises. Criteria are then used to diagnosis diabetes or the less severe IGT (Expert Committee, 2003). **Gestational diabetes mellitus** occurs in a small percentage of women during pregnancy. It usually ends after the pregnancy, but women who experience GDM have a high risk of developing type 2 diabetes later in life.

Exercise therapy for clients with type 1 diabetes is aimed primarily at reducing the risk of cardiovascular disease and improving overall fitness. Exercise therapy for clients with type 2 diabetes is potentially a very effective treatment for the disease itself. Because exercise training improves insulin sensitivity (Devlin, 1992), people with type 2 diabetes who exercise sufficiently often can normalize their blood glucose control. In one research study, five people with type 2 diabetes and eight people with IGT entered a one-year exercise program (Holloszy et al., 1986). Over the year, they built up their exercise time to 50 to 60 minutes, five times per week, at 70 to 90% of maximal $\dot{V}O_2$. At the end of the year, three of the five patients with diabetes and all eight of the IGT patients had completely normalized their responses to glucose tolerance tests. (Note that many of the IGT patients in this 1986 study might be classified as having type 2 diabetes today, because the criterion for diagnosing diabetes mellitus from fasting glucose was >140 mg $\cdot$ dl^{-1} then.) Although exercise is highly effective at improving insulin sensitivity, like any fitness adaptation, the improved sensitivity regresses if regular exercise is not maintained (Albright et al., 2000).

EXERCISE PRESCRIPTION FOR CLIENTS WITH TYPE 1 DIABETES

You can use the standard ACSM exercise prescription guidelines for clients with either type 1 or type 2 diabetes (see table 2.1). However, people with diabetes are in the ACSM's high-risk category and should be evaluated by a physician before starting an exercise program. "Medical Evaluation of Clients with Diabetes Prior to Exercise" lists common secondary complications of diabetes that should be considered in the medical evaluation (ACSM, 2006; American Diabetes Association, 2000).

Once people with diabetes enter an exercise program, they should take special care to avoid hypoglycemia—a risk particularly for those with type 1 diabetes. Because both insulin and exercise reduce blood glucose, there is the potential for a dangerous fall in blood glucose during and after exercise. Clients with type 1 diabetes who have a planned exercise routine should reduce the insulin dosage of the pre-exercise injection. Although people differ widely in their responses, a good starting point is to reduce the short-acting insulin taken prior to exercise by 30 to 50% (Colberg, 2000; Colberg and Swain, 2000). Alternatively, they can increase carbohydrate intake prior to exercise.

Although planning ahead is preferable, people inevitably decide on impulse to go out for a run or a game of tennis. People with type 1 diabetes who are about to engage in unplanned exercise should consider consuming 20 to 30 g of carbohydrates for each 30 minutes of anticipated exercise to prevent a fall in blood glucose during the exercise. Everyone with diabetes, regardless of the type, should have a fast-acting source of sugar (e.g., juice, hard candy) available during exercise to consume immediately if hypoglycemic symptoms occur (e.g., weakness, light-headedness). Hypoglycemia requires immediate attention, because it can quickly become life-threatening. One or two pieces of hard candy or a small glass of juice should relieve symptoms in less than five minutes. If someone loses consciousness, call 911 or whatever the emergency number is in your area. Prior to the arrival of emergency personnel, try squirting a sugar-containing gel (or even cake frosting) onto the

Medical Evaluation of Clients With Diabetes Prior to Exercise

Metabolic Control

The person must have an acceptable level of glucose control (<300 mg · dl^{-1}, preferably <250 mg · dl^{-1}), through medication if needed, because exercise can worsen hyperglycemia.

Coronary Artery Disease

Given the increased risk caused by diabetes, people with diabetes who are older than 35, and those who have additional risk factors, should have a stress test. Beta-blockers may mask symptoms of hypoglycemia.

Retinopathy

If proliferative retinopathy or moderate to severe nonproliferative retinopathy is present, the person must avoid exercises that jar the body or that induce a hypertensive response. Those who have undergone laser treatment must obtain approval of an ophthalmologist before proceeding with an exercise program.

Autonomic Neuropathy

Assess all clients with diabetes for orthostatic intolerance and use seated exercise if needed. Clients with diabetic autonomic neuropathy (DAN) have a blunted HR response to exercise (i.e., HR does not rise as much as otherwise expected). Clients with DAN should avoid exercise in excessive heat.

Peripheral Neuropathy

Clients with peripheral neuropathy should clean and examine their feet regularly. Consider non-weight-bearing exercise for clients with this condition.

Nephropathy

Exercise capacity may be reduced in clients with nephropathy. Thus, exercise intensity should be low.

inner surface of the unconscious person's cheek. Following are steps clients can take before, during, and after exercise to avoid hypoglycemia (ACSM, 2006; American Diabetes Association, 2000; Colberg, 2000).

Steps to Avoid Hypoglycemia*

Prior to Planned Exercise

Reduce pre-exercise insulin (based on individual responsiveness).

Prior to Unplanned Exercise

Consume 20 to 30 g of carbohydrates (insulin users only for each 30 min of anticipated exercise).

Prior to Any Exercise

Consume 20 to 30 g of carbohydrates if blood glucose <100 mg · dl^{-1}.

During Exercise

Consume 20 to 30 g of carbohydrates each 30 min for extended exercise (insulin users only).
Be aware of symptoms of hypoglycemia.
Exercise with a partner.
Carry fast-acting sugar and consume as needed if hypoglycemia occurs.

After Exercise

Consume 20 to 30 g of carbohydrates if blood glucose <100 mg · dl^{-1}.
Be aware of the potential for hypoglycemia for several hours.

*Note: These are guidelines only. They must be adapted to clients on an individual basis.

Exercise can exacerbate hyperglycemia and ketosis. To minimize the risk of either hyper- or hypoglycemia, patients should monitor their blood glucose frequently at the start of a new exercise program. They should check blood glucose immediately before exercise and evaluate it using the information in table 9.1 (ACSM, 2006; American Diabetes Association 2000). They should also check it after exercise: If it is rising, they should consult their physician. A rising blood glucose suggests that the patient may need an insulin injection, *to be determined by the physician,* to prevent ketosis and a possible diabetic coma. This is a much rarer consequence of exercise than is hypoglycemia, but both you and the patients with whom you work should be aware of the possibility. However, also be aware that glucose could rise as a result of the consumption of carbohydrates during the exercise or as a result of a sympathetic response to intense exercise. In general, the postexercise value

Table 9.1 Interpreting Blood Glucose Values Prior to Exercise

If >300 mg · dl⁻¹	Postpone exercise; consult physician/inject insulin.
If >250 mg · dl⁻¹	Check for urinary ketones; if present, postpone exercise, consult physician/inject insulin.
If 100-250 mg · dl⁻¹	OK to begin exercise.
If <100 mg · dl⁻¹	Consume 20-30 g of carbohydrates prior to exercising.

should be no more than the pre-exercise value. Some decrease is normal, but if it has fallen much more than is typical for that particular person, or has fallen below 100 mg · dl⁻¹, the person should consume extra carbohydrates.

With proper attention to the details of glucose and insulin management, people with type 1 diabetes can enjoy vigorous athletic pursuits (Colberg, 2000).

CASE STUDY 9.1
Client With Type 1 Diabetes Mellitus

Sheri is a 17-year-old high school distance runner. Over the past few weeks she began experiencing a number of unusual symptoms. The first symptom she noticed was that she had to get up during the night to urinate, eventually having to do this several times each night. She became thirsty all the time, even though she drank lots of water. She started losing weight and at the same time experienced an increase in her appetite. It seemed that no matter how much she ate, she still kept losing weight. Furthermore, her workouts were suffering. She felt constantly tired and lethargic, and her performance times were worsening even though she continued her regular training. Her family physician found her blood glucose to be 380 mg · dl⁻¹. The physician diagnosed her with type 1 diabetes mellitus and placed her on a twice-daily regimen of insulin injections, each injection consisting of both intermediate-acting (NPH) and short-acting (Humalog) insulin. Over the three months since her diagnosis, Sheri has experienced several bouts of hypoglycemia, and her physician has modified her insulin dosage until her glucose levels have become fairly stable. During this time, she has been prohibited from running. She is now ready to resume her running, and her physician has referred her to you for advice and an exercise prescription. Her resting HR is 56 bpm, and her maximal HR measured during training is 194 bpm.

Sheri needs to return *gradually* to her former competitive training level, as would anyone coming back from a three-month layoff. You prescribe three exercise sessions per week at the beginning, on alternate days. Her previous training runs were over an hour long, but your initial prudent goal is 30 minutes. You set her intensity at a moderate level, which she is probably very capable of judging by her personal feelings of perceived exertion. However, to keep her from overdoing it at first, you provide a target HR range at 50 to 70% of HRR. Her maximal HR is 194 bpm, so use that value in the calculation of target HR, rather than 220 − age.

$$\text{Target HR} = (\text{intensity fraction})(\text{HRmax} - \text{HRrest}) + \text{HRrest}$$

$$\text{Lower target HR} = 0.50(194 - 56) + 56$$

$$= 0.50(138) + 56$$

$$= 69 + 56$$

$$= 125 \text{ bpm}$$

$$\text{Upper target HR} = 0.70(19.4 - 56) + 56$$

$$= 0.70(138) + 56$$

$$= 97 + 56$$

$$= 153 \text{ bpm}$$

Sheri should already be monitoring her blood glucose several times a day. If she is not, she needs to now. Ask her to measure her blood glucose when she wakes up. If the reading is her typical morning value, she should take her morning (prebreakfast) insulin injection, but she should reduce the dosage of short-acting insulin (Humalog) by 50% if she plans to exercise within one to two hours. If her exercise session will be in the afternoon, she should reduce the intermediate-acting insulin (NPH) instead, which does not reach peak levels in the bloodstream for at least four hours.

After her usual breakfast, Sheri should wait about an hour before starting preparations for her first run. Immediately before

(continued)

Case Study 9.1 *(continued)*

the run, she should measure her blood glucose again. During the run, she should carry a fast-acting sugar source and pay attention to possible symptoms of hypoglycemia. Inform her that exercise can mask or change her usual hypoglycemic symptoms. Until her pattern is well established, she may need to arrange to check her blood glucose level halfway through her run as well.

After the run, Sheri should measure her blood glucose again, and if necessary, consume a carbohydrate snack at that time. If her postexercise blood glucose is less than 100 mg $\cdot$ dl^{-1}, or if she experiences any symptoms of hypoglycemia during or closely following her run, ask her to further reduce her preexercise insulin dosage for the exercise session two days from now. If her postexercise glucose is higher than her preexercise glucose, she will need to moderate the reduction in preexercise insulin. Instruct her to pay close attention to the possible development of hypoglycemia over the next couple of hours leading up to lunch time and even up to 24 hours after her running while she is unaccustomed to it. If she experiences nocturnal bouts of hypoglycemia following training days, then she will need to reduce her evening dose of intermediate-acting insulin (NPH) as well or consume an additional bedtime snack to compensate.

Sheri also needs to be aware of several other effects from regular training: (1) Her overall insulin needs may decrease with her regular activity, and she may need to reduce her intermediate-acting insulin (NPH) in addition to reducing her short-acting insulin (Humalog) during the training season if her food intake does not increase enough to compensate. (2) Training can increase her body's ability to use fat as fuel, and her blood sugars may begin to drop less during an activity once she has become accustomed to it. (3) Successive days of heavy exercise increase her risk for hypoglycemia, especially during the night. She may need to monitor her blood glucose levels during the night in this case, adjust her evening insulin doses, or eat an additional snack at bedtime.

You can help Sheri fine-tune her insulin regimen as she increases her training frequency, duration, and intensity back to her previous level. It is critical for her to recognize the importance of balancing a regular regimen of training with changes in insulin and diet to accomplish this successfully.

EXERCISE PRESCRIPTION FOR CLIENTS WITH TYPE 2 DIABETES

The principal goal for prescribing exercise for clients with type 2 diabetes is to burn calories. Most people with type 2 diabetes are obese, and burning calories attacks the diabetes twice: first, by improving tissue sensitivity to insulin; and second, by reducing body fat. The exercise prescription therefore should focus on increasing the duration and frequency of exercise, using an intensity level that the client can sustain for long periods of time. For best results, clients should gradually increase the duration and frequency to one hour, seven days per week. Two 30-minute sessions per day or three 20-minute sessions are perfectly acceptable ways to accomplish the same goal. Use these same guidelines to prescribe exercise for people with impaired fasting glucose or impaired glucose tolerance. Women with gestational diabetes also need an exercise prescription that focuses on calorie burning, but this must be tempered as needed with the concerns associated with pregnancy itself (see chapter 10).

Because most clients with type 2 diabetes start out with a low fitness level, prescribe light to moderate exercise intensity (e.g., 40 to 60% of $\dot{V}O_2R$). A greater intensity will burn more calories, but it is less likely to be sustained long enough to burn as many calories as a more moderate intensity. Moreover, high-intensity programs may lead to a greater dropout rate than those requiring only moderate intensities. Despite the drawbacks of high-intensity prescriptions, however, it is still a good idea to encourage clients to increase the intensity *within their level of tolerance* as their programs progress.

Clients with type 2 diabetes are much less likely than those with type 1 diabetes to experience either hypoglycemia or hyperglycemia as a result of exercise. The exception is type 2 clients who take insulin: Their responses are much more like those with type 1 diabetes, and you should handle them accordingly. Hypoglycemia is comparatively rare with type 2 diabetes, but be sure that all such clients are aware of its potential, remain alert to its symptoms, and carry a fast-acting source of sugar during exercise.

People with type 2 diabetes are just as susceptible as those with type 1 to the secondary complications listed in "Medical

Evaluation of Clients With Diabetes Prior to Exercise" on page 132. It is imperative that they be evaluated by a physician prior to starting an exercise program.

CASE STUDY 9.2
Client With Type 2 Diabetes Mellitus

Rudy is 72 years old, 5'10" tall, and weighs 287 lb. He was diagnosed with type 2 diabetes five years ago and has been treated with oral hypoglycemic agents. His physician has told him that he must do a better job with diet and exercise, or eventually he will have to go on insulin. He gets no regular exercise, and his diet consists largely of red meats, fried foods, and creamy sauces. At his last medical checkup, Rudy had a total cholesterol of 264 mg · dl^{-1}; his LDL was 145 mg · dl^{-1}, his HDL was 38 mg · dl^{-1}, and his fasting glucose was 156 mg · dl^{-1}. Because of his high risk of heart disease, he was given a stress test. He completed a cycling protocol up to 140 W, obtaining a maximal HR of 160 bpm. His resting HR is 78 bpm. There were no signs of coronary ischemia. His physician reports that he has no other overt medical conditions at this time and has referred him to your facility for lifestyle modification and an exercise prescription. Rudy rarely monitors his blood sugar. He says strips are too expensive.

Rudy is quite typical of people with type 2 diabetes. He is obese (BMI of 41 kg · m^{-2}), has elevated LDL (and total) cholesterol, is sedentary, and has only moderate control over his blood glucose levels. These factors all greatly increase his risk of heart disease. Fortunately, he does not yet exhibit clinically significant heart disease. Encourage him to set a goal of reaching a target weight at a BMI of 25 kg · m^{-2}, which would be about 174 lb. Losing approximately 110 lb of fat will take one year of consistent exercise and dietary discipline. He should reduce his caloric intake by about 500 kcal per day, primarily through selecting foods that are lower in fat than those he currently chooses.

You begin his exercise prescription with 20-minute sessions, three times per week, at 40 to 60% of $\dot{V}O_2R$. You can use a target HR range or a target workload to establish the intensity. Over the next few weeks, he needs to increase the frequency and duration of his exercise to an effective level (i.e., to one hour daily if he is willing). Your primary task is to convince Rudy of the value of performing this much exercise. His target HR would be as follows:

$$\text{Target HR} = (\text{intensity fraction})(\text{HRmax} - \text{HRrest}) + \text{HRrest}$$

$$\text{Lower target HR} = (0.40)(160 - 78) + 78$$

$$= (0.40)(82) + 78$$

$$= 33 + 78$$

$$= 111 \text{ bpm}$$

$$\text{Upper target HR} = (0.60)(160 - 78) + 78$$

$$= (0.60)(82) + 78$$

$$= 49 + 78$$

$$= 127 \text{ bpm}$$

You could determine his target workload by (1) estimating his $\dot{V}O_2$max from his maximal workload of 140 W; (2) determining the target $\dot{V}O_2$ at 40 to 60% of $\dot{V}O_2$R; and then (3) converting the target $\dot{V}O_2$ into the target workload. A simple approximation would be to just take 40 to 60% of the maximal workload itself:

$$\text{Lower target workload} = (0.40)(140 \text{ W})$$

$$= 56 \text{ W}$$

$$\text{Upper target workload} = (0.60)(140 \text{ W})$$

$$= 84 \text{ W}$$

Thus, you gauge his exercise intensity as a HR between 111 and 127 bpm or as a workload between 56 and 84 W. To determine a workload on a piece of equipment that does not indicate the power in watts, such as a treadmill, you would need to go through the three steps listed earlier for converting to a $\dot{V}O_2$ and then back to a workload.

How many net calories will Rudy burn with his exercise program? Using the 84 W ($84 \times 6 = 504 \text{ kg} \cdot \text{m} \cdot \text{min}^{-1}$) workload at

(continued)

his current body weight of 287 lb (287 / 2.2 =130.5 kg), you obtain the following:

$$\dot{V}O_2 = 7 + 1.8(\text{workload}) / (\text{body mass})$$

$$= 7 + 1.8(504) / 130.5$$

$$= 7 + 907.2 / 130.5$$

$$= 7 + 7.0$$

$$= 14 \text{ ml} \cdot \text{min}^{-1} \cdot \text{kg}^{-1}$$

$$\text{Net } \dot{V}O_2 = 14 - 3.5 = 10.5 \text{ ml} \cdot \text{min}^{-1} \cdot \text{kg}^{-1}$$

$$\frac{(10.5 \text{ ml} \cdot \text{min}^{-1} \cdot \text{kg}^{-1}) (130.5 \text{ kg})}{1,000} = 1.37 \text{ L} \cdot \text{min}^{-1}$$

$$(1.37 \text{ L} \cdot \text{min}^{-1}) \times 5 = 6.85 \text{ kcal} \cdot \text{min}^{-1}$$

If Rudy burns a net 6.85 kcal per minute for 30 minutes, three times a week, this would total 6.85 × 30 × 3 = 617 kcal per week. There are 3,500 kcal stored in a pound of fat, so he would be losing less than one-fifth of a pound per week through the exercise (617 / 3,500 = 0.18 lb). However, if he does his exercises for 60 minutes, seven times per week, it would total 6.85 × 60 × 7 = 2,877 kcal per week. This is a little more than four-fifths of a pound of fat each week (2,877 / 3,500 = 0.82 lb). He has also been asked to reduce his caloric intake by 500 kcal per day (i.e., 3,500 kcal, or 1 lb per week), so he should be losing nearly 2 lb per week with this program. Be sure to reevaluate his status every three months and modify his program as appropriate. Although at some point in the future you should consider incorporating resistance training into his program, for the time being Rudy needs to focus his available time on burning calories.

Rudy is reluctant to monitor his blood glucose, in part because of the financial cost. It is imperative, however, that he monitor his blood glucose before and after each exercise session when he first begins the program. Once he establishes a steady response pattern, it would be acceptable for him to reduce his monitoring to one exercise session per week. However, as with all patients with diabetes, *it would be better if he would monitor several times daily.*

As his condition improves, his current level of hypoglycemic medication may be too much. He will need to be aware of the growing possibility of hypoglycemia, and his physician will probably have to reduce his medication as the year progresses. It is quite possible that he will be able to get off his medication entirely.

CASE STUDY 9.3
Type 2 Client With Secondary Complications

Juanita is 56 years old, 5'1" tall, and weighs 192 lb. She was diagnosed with type 2 diabetes at age 38 and has injected insulin twice daily for the past seven years. She has had ulcers on her feet that are currently healed, and she has been diagnosed with peripheral neuropathy. She has moderate nonproliferative retinopathy. She was given an arm ergometry stress test recently, and her $\dot{V}O_2$max was measured at 11 ml·min⁻¹·kg⁻¹, with a maximal HR of 152 bpm. Her resting HR is 92 bpm. She exhibited 2 mm of ST depression at maximal exercise but no abnormal heart rhythms or symptoms of ischemia. On follow-up, an angiogram revealed mild blockage of two coronary arteries—for which she currently takes aspirin and beta-blockers. She has been referred to your facility for exercise training.

In creating an exercise prescription for Juanita, you need to consider the secondary complications of her diabetes.

Peripheral neuropathy: She has poor sensation in her feet, and she will need to inspect and clean her feet at least once a day and immediately after each exercise session. She may need to select exercises that require her feet to bear less weight, based on her level of tolerance. Walking is a possibility, but she may have to use stationary cycling or rowing or possibly even arm ergometry.

Retinopathy: Juanita must avoid exercises that entail jarring or large increases in blood pressure. Jarring should not be a problem because you are already limiting her weight-bearing exercises because of her foot problems. To avoid excessive increases in blood pressure, instruct her to avoid the Valsalva maneuver during resistance training and to consider using a lighter weight that she can lift 10 to 15 times without going to failure.

(continued)

Case Study 9.3   *(continued)*

Coronary heart disease: Because Juanita performed her stress test before she was placed on beta-blockers, you can't use the HR data that were collected at that time to establish target HRs. If she does another stress test while on her medication, you can use that information to determine target HRs, because the HR response to exercise under beta-blockade is still linear. For the time being, use RPE or target workload to establish intensity. Begin her exercise prescription at 40 to 60% of $\dot{V}O_2R$ for 20 to 30 minutes, three times per week. Table 3.1 shows that an intensity of 40 to 60% of $\dot{V}O_2R$ corresponds to an RPE of 12 to 14. Target workloads using arm ergometry are calculated here.

$$\text{Target } \dot{V}O_2 = (\text{intensity fraction})(\dot{V}O_2\text{max} - 3.5) + 3.5$$

$$\text{Lower target } \dot{V}O_2 = (0.40)(11 - 3.5) + 3.5$$

$$= (0.40)(7.5) + 3.5$$

$$= 3.0 + 3.5$$

$$= 6.5 \text{ ml} \cdot \text{min}^{-1} \cdot \text{kg}^{-1}$$

$$\text{Upper target } \dot{V}O_2 = (0.60)(11 - 3.5) + 3.5$$

$$= (0.60)(7.5) + 3.5$$

$$= 4.5 + 3.5$$

$$= 8.0 \text{ ml} \cdot \text{min}^{-1} \cdot \text{kg}^{-1}$$

Now, determine the corresponding workloads on an arm ergometer.

$$\dot{V}O_2 = 3.5 + 3(\text{work rate}) / (\text{body mass})$$

Lower target workload:

$$6.5 = 3.5 + 3(\text{work rate}) / 87.3$$

$$6.5 - 3.5 = 3(\text{work rate}) / 87.3$$

$$3.0 = 3(\text{work rate}) / 87.3$$

$$3/3 = (\text{work rate}) / 87.3$$

$$1.0 = (\text{work rate})/87.3$$

$$87.3 \text{ kg} \cdot \text{m} \cdot \text{min}^{-1} = \text{work rate}$$

Upper target workload:

$$8.0 = 3.5 + 3(\text{work rate}) / 87.3$$

$$8.0 - 3.5 = 3(\text{work rate}) / 87.3$$

$$4.5 = 3(\text{work rate}) / 87.3$$

$$4.5/3 = (\text{work rate}) / 87.3$$

$$1.5 = (\text{work rate}) / 87.3$$

$$1.5 \times 87.3 = \text{work rate}$$

$$131 \text{ kg} \cdot \text{m} \cdot \text{min}^{-1} = \text{work rate}$$

What would be the resistance setting if Juanita uses a Monark arm ergometer (2.4 m flywheel distance) at a cadence of 50 rpm? Use the cycle ergometry work rate equation from chapter 4.

Work rate = (resistance setting)(flywheel distance per rev)(rpm)

Lower target workload:

$$87 = (\text{resistance setting})(2.4)(50)$$

$$87 = (\text{resistance setting})(120)$$

$$87 / 120 = \text{resistance setting}$$

$$0.73 \text{ kg} = \text{resistance setting}$$

Upper target workload:

$$131 = (\text{resistance setting})(120)$$

$$131 / 120 = \text{resistance setting}$$

$$1.09 \text{ kg} = \text{resistance setting}$$

Juanita should use a resistance setting of about 0.7 to 1.1 kg on the arm ergometer if she is cranking at 50 rpm.

Juanita is obese (BMI of 36 kg $\cdot$ m^{-2}) and would benefit from a structured weight loss program. Because she uses insulin, you will need to increase the frequency and duration of her exercise very carefully. Like Sheri, the teenage girl with type 1 diabetes in case study 9.1, Juanita will need to reduce her preexercise insulin dosage and pay special attention to the risk of hypoglycemia during exercise.

REFERENCES

ACSM. 2006. *ACSM's Guidelines for Exercise Testing and Prescription*, 7th ed., 207-211. Philadelphia: Lippincott Williams & Wilkins.

Albright, A., M. Franz, G. Hornsby, A. Kriska, D. Marrero, I. Ullrich, and L.S. Verity. 2000. Exercise and type 2 diabetes (ACSM position stand). *Medicine and Science in Sports and Exercise* 32: 1345-1360.

American Diabetes Association. 2000. Diabetes mellitus and exercise—position statement. *Diabetes Care* 23 (Suppl. 1): S50-54.

Colberg, S.R. 2000. *The Diabetic Athlete*. Champaign, IL: Human Kinetics.

Colberg S.R., and D.P. Swain. 2000. Exercise and diabetes control. *Physician and Sportsmedicine* 28 (4): 63-81.

Devlin, J.T. 1992. Effects of exercise on insulin sensitivity in humans. *Diabetes Care* 15: 1690-1693.

Expert Committee. 2003. Report of the Expert Committee on the diagnosis and classification of diabetes mellitus. *Diabetes Care* 26: S5-S20.

Holloszy, J.O., J. Schultz, J. Kusnierkiewicz, J.M. Hagberg, and A.A. Ehsani. 1986. Effect of exercise on glucose tolerance and insulin resistance. *Acta Medica Scandinavica* (Suppl.) 711: 55-65.

C H A P T E R

10

Exercise Prescription for Other Special Cases

This chapter discusses ACSM exercise prescriptions for a variety of special cases, some of which are clinical conditions that can appear in the same patient: peripheral arterial disease (PAD), chronic obstructive pulmonary disease (COPD), and hypertension (HTN). In addition, it covers the special cases of exercise during pregnancy and exercise prescription for children.

PERIPHERAL ARTERIAL DISEASE

Peripheral arterial disease (PAD), sometimes referred to as **peripheral vascular disease (PVD),** is a condition that results in occlusion or blockage of the arteries of the lower extremities. This results in insufficient blood flow, lactic acid accumulation, and a burning pain in the affected muscles (known as claudication), such as the calves. Ten percent of adults over 70 years of age have signs or symptoms of PAD. This condition affects approximately 8 to 10 million people in the United States. Many people with PAD are so deconditioned that they depend on others to perform routine tasks, such as walking to the end of their driveway to get the daily mail.

The goals for PAD exercise programs are to improve patients' walking ability, reduce associated atherosclerotic risks, and improve their tolerance to calf pain. Many patients with PAD also have coronary artery disease and are therefore at high risk and should have an exercise test prior to beginning an exercise program. The exercise test should be performed on a cycle ergometer to rule out associated coronary artery disease, or on a treadmill to diagnose PAD or baseline walking ability, and the onset of claudication pain. Despite the fact that most people with PAD avoid walking activities, walking should be the primary mode of exercise to improve circulation in the legs. A patient limited by claudication should initially perform intermittent exercise, in which she walks until the pain becomes intense enough that she cannot be distracted from it (level 3 out of 4 in the "Claudication Scale"). After resting until the pain dissipates, the patient repeats the walk/rest intervals until she has completed at least 35 minutes, and up to 50 minutes, of actual walking. Once the patient can perform at least 20 minutes of continuous walking, then standard use of the FITT principle may be employed, consistent with exercise prescription for coronary heart disease patients in chapter 8. Resistance training may be added to the PAD patient's regimen as tolerated.

Claudication Scale

Grade 1   Minimal pain or discomfort

Grade 2   Moderate pain or discomfort, but attention can be diverted

Grade 3   Intense pain, attention cannot be diverted

Grade 4   Excruciating pain, cannot continue

Adapted, by permission, from American College of Sports Medicine (ACSM), 2006, *ACSM's guidelines for exercise testing and prescription*, 7th ed. (Philadelphia, PA: Lippincott Williams & Wilkins), 107.

CASE STUDY 10.1

Client With Peripheral Arterial Disease

Juan is a 60-year-old male who suffers from peripheral arterial disease (PAD) and moderate chronic obstructive pulmonary disease (COPD). He has been unsuccessful in smoking cessation programs and currently smokes between one and two packs of cigarettes per day. Many people with PAD smoke, and Juan's history of smoking has probably resulted in his COPD. During a treadmill test, Juan could walk at only 2 mph for 30 seconds when he developed severe, burning leg pain in his calf that forced him to stop. Doppler studies revealed an ankle-to-arm pressure index less than 0.90 at rest (i.e., ankle systolic BP is less than 90% of brachial systolic BP). He was then given an arm ergometer test. Results of this test were as follows:

- **ECG:** Normal sinus rhythm
- **Peak heart rate:** 130 bpm
- **Resting heart rate:** 75 bpm
- **Peak blood pressure:** 148/92 mmHg
- **Resting blood pressure:** 128/86 mmHg
- **S_aO_2 at peak exercise:** 93%
- **Peak work rate:** 60 W

Whenever a person presents with more than one chronic condition, you should focus the exercise prescription on the most severe condition. Juan's PAD is significant (though not in the "severe" range), based on his pain during walking and his poor ankle-to-arm systolic index. His COPD is less significant, because his arterial oxygen saturation (S_aO_2) does not drop below 88% during exercise. Therefore, because his ability to exercise is limited by his PAD and not his COPD, focus Juan's exercise prescription on his PAD using the FITT principle and following ACSM recommendations.

Frequency: The frequency of exercise should be at least three days per week. However, people who can exercise only intermittently and at low intensity should exercise every day to maximize improvements.

Intensity: An intensity of 40 to 70% of $\dot{V}O_2$max is recommended. Note that the ACSM has changed the basis for cardiorespiratory exercise prescription from %$\dot{V}O_2$max to %$\dot{V}O_2$R for most situations; however, it has still retained the terminology of %$\dot{V}O_2$max for certain special populations. In Juan's case, exercise prescription based on $\dot{V}O_2$ would be appropriate only for arm exercise, because his HR and $\dot{V}O_2$ responses to leg exercise are not known. The peak HR and $\dot{V}O_2$ during arm exercise are generally much less than during leg exercise. When performing leg exercises, Juan should exercise until he reaches a pain level of 3 out of 4 on the claudication scale and then rest until he is able to resume exercise. In this way, he will be able to increase his exercise tolerance.

(continued)

Case Study 10.1 *(continued)*

Time: You prescribe 35 to 50 minutes of accumulated exercise per session. You tell Juan that he need not achieve this amount in one continuous exercise bout, but he may perform multiple discontinuous bouts as his comfort level permits.

Type: You recommend weight-bearing exercise such as walking to improve circulation in Juan's lower limbs. However, you point out that he can extend his exercise session by replacing rest periods with non-weight-bearing activities such as cycling, swimming, or arm ergometry. In this way he can maintain the intensity and increase the duration of his exercise, thereby improving his cardiovascular fitness.

To conclude the case study, assume that Juan has progressed and is now able to do 20 minutes of continuous exercise and can complete a treadmill exercise test. This is an important milestone, because his earlier arm ergometry test may not have reached a high enough intensity to reveal underlying heart disease. You are now able to measure his cardiorespiratory fitness and can prescribe exercise using a target heart rate (HR). His maximal heart rate is 150 bpm, achieved by walking 2 mph at a 10% grade. Metabolic data are not available. Calculate a target HR range for Juan using the percent heart rate reserve (%HRR) method. First, calculate his $\dot{V}O_2$max using the walking equation from page 50 to determine the appropriate intensity level to apply to his target HR range. His walking speed is 2 mph $\times$ 26.8 = 53.6 m · min^{-1}.

$$\dot{V}O_2 = 3.5 + 0.1(\text{speed}) + 1.8(\text{speed})(\text{fractional grade})$$

$$= 3.5 + 0.1(53.6) + 1.8(53.6)(0.10)$$

$$= 3.5 + 5.36 + 9.648$$

$$= 18.5 \text{ ml · } min^{-1} \cdot kg^{-1}$$

Juan's aerobic capacity is low. Using the formula in table 4.1 ($\dot{V}O_2$ in ml · min^{-1} · kg^{-1} / 3.5 = $\dot{V}O_2$ in METs), we see that it is only 18.5 ml · min^{-1} · kg^{-1} / 3.5 = 5.3 METs. You therefore use a heart rate range of 40 to 60%. Juan's resting heart rate is 75 bpm.

Target HR = (intensity fraction)(HRmax − HRrest) + HRrest

Lower target HR = (0.40)(150 − 75) + 75

= (0.40)(75) + 75

= 30 + 75

= 105 bpm

Upper target HR = (0.60)(150 − 75) + 75

= (0.60)(75) + 75

= 45 + 75

= 120 bpm

CHRONIC OBSTRUCTIVE PULMONARY DISEASE

Chronic obstructive pulmonary disease (COPD) is common in cigarette smokers and consists of emphysema, chronic bronchitis, or a combination of the two. Obstructive pulmonary disease refers to an increased airway resistance that is most noticeable on exhalation; clinically, this is detected as a decrease in FEV_1 (the volume of air that can be exhaled in one second). COPD patients experience difficulty in breathing (dyspnea) that is first noticed during exercise, but which often progresses to the point that breathing is labored even at rest. The benefits of exercise for individuals with COPD include increased exercise capacity, functional status, and quality of life, as well as a decrease in the severity of dyspnea. Individuals who have COPD or other lung diseases generally experience a gradual downhill prognosis. Rather than attempting to reverse the disease, exercise-based rehabilitation should aim to reduce the functional impairment. Oxygen saturation levels should be monitored during exercise, and oxygen should be administered if levels fall below 88%.

Another obstructive disorder is asthma, characterized by a sudden increase in airway resistance as a result of constriction of the bronchioles. This bronchoconstriction may be caused by an allergic reaction to inhaled irritants (such as pollen); certain foods in sensitive individuals; or cold, dry air. Bronchoconstriction from cold, dry air often occurs during exercise, when air flow increases, and is referred to as exercise-induced asthma (EIA). When asthma is well controlled, by the avoidance of irritants and the use of prophylactic drugs (such as albuterol administered via an inhaler), it is possible to prescribe exercise using the standard principles outlined in chapter 3.

For COPD patients, walking is the recommended mode of exercise, three to five days per week. The intensity of exercise should be prescribed based on individual limitations. The ACSM recommends the use of either 50% of peak $\dot{V}O_2$ or an intensity that evokes mild to moderate, but not severe, dyspnea (i.e., 2 or 3 on the 4-point dyspnea scale on page 151). The exercise prescription for resistance training should be individualized to the patient's ability.

CASE STUDY 10.2

Client With Chronic Obstructive Pulmonary Disease

Penelope is 60 years old, with a lifelong history of cigarette smoking. She has severe chronic obstructive pulmonary disease (COPD), and her S_aO_2 falls below 88% when she exercises. She has been admitted to your pulmonary rehabilitation program for exercise conditioning.

Using the FITT principle and ACSM recommendations (ACSM, 2006), you devise Penelope's exercise prescription as follows:

Frequency: Most COPD exercise programs are hospital based and range from one to five days per week, averaging two days, usually Tuesdays and Thursdays. Patients who are "end-stage" may be inconsistent in their ability to exercise. Therefore, you must consider patient variability and functional status when determining the frequency.

Intensity: Penelope desaturates during exercise, so it is important to use a pulse oximeter to monitor her arterial oxygen S_aO_2 to prevent it from falling below 88%. Should her S_aO_2 regularly fall below 88% when she is exercising at her prescribed intensity, you need to decrease the intensity and contact her physician. You may want to request that her physician prescribe a nasal oxygen cannula for Penelope to use during exercise. If metabolic data are available for Penelope, you may want to prescribe her exercise at 50% of peak oxygen consumption. More likely, you will need to prescribe her intensity based on her symptoms. Like Juan, the PAD patient in case study 10.1, she should exercise up to her level of tolerance and try to increase the duration of her intermittent bouts. One means of gauging her intensity would be by the use of a dyspnea scale, of which there are several. As an example, she could attempt to work at level 3 on the Dyspnea scale:

Dyspnea Scale

+1 Mild, noticeable to patient but not observer

+2 Mild, some difficulty, noticeable to observer

+3 Moderate difficulty, but can continue

+4 Severe difficulty, cannot continue

Adapted, by permission, from American College of Sports Medicine (ACSM), 2006, *ACSM's guidelines for exercise testing and prescription*, 7th ed. (Philadelphia, PA: Lippincott Williams & Wilkins), 107.

Time: Continuous exercise of 20 minutes or more would be desirable. However, as with PAD, accumulating this much time through repeated bouts of intermittent exercise is more appropriate for most patients, until they are able to tolerate continuous exercise.

Type: You should prescribe aerobic activities that involve large muscle activities such as walking, cycling, and swimming. Aerobic exercise that focuses on smaller muscle groups, such as arm ergometry, may result in a higher ventilation and may not be tolerated as well. You also will want to add strength training two or three days per week, especially for the upper body, using low resistance and high repetitions.

Instruct Penelope in pursed-lips breathing (i.e., she should inhale through her nose and exhale through a small gap between her lips). Because exhaling in this manner extends the time of the exhalation and requires more force, it potentially can keep airways more open. Penelope should use pursed-lips breathing not only during exercise but whenever she experiences dyspnea.

HYPERTENSION

Hypertension (HTN) is a major health problem in the United States and other Western industrialized countries. It has been estimated that there are as many as 50 million Americans and one billion individuals worldwide with high blood pressure, many of whom are taking medications. **Hypertension** is defined as systolic blood pressure consistently above 140 mmHg or a diastolic blood pressure consistently above 90 mmHg. High blood pressure is classified into two categories, primary (or essential) and secondary. Approximately 95% of individuals with hypertension have **primary hypertension,** in which the cause is not apparent. The remaining 5% have **secondary hypertension,** due to endocrine or renal abnormalities. Although primary hypertension has no known direct cause, it is related to a variety of factors including inactivity, obesity, alcohol intake, and (in sodium-sensitive individuals) salt intake.

Regular aerobic exercise can play an important role in reducing elevated blood pressure and should be prescribed following an exercise test. Individuals training aerobically at 40 to 70% of their HRR or $\dot{V}O_2R$, three to seven days per week, for 30 to 60 minutes have demonstrated a 5 to 7 mmHg reduction in blood pressure (Fagard, 2001). Patients with resting blood pressures that exceed 200/110 should not exercise; during exercise testing, if blood pressures exceed 250/115, the test should be terminated. (Note that the ACSM *Guidelines* use 260 mmHg as the cutoff in the chapter on hypertension but use 250 mmHg as the cutoff in both chapters on exercise testing; ACSM, 2006.) Resistance training should incorporate low resistance and high repetitions, but only in individuals who have stable and controlled hypertension. Because of the type of medications patients are on, postexercise hypotension may result. Therefore, extended cool-down times are recommended.

CASE STUDY 10.3
Client With Hypertension

Collin has a history of hypertension that is currently managed by his physician with beta-blockers. Collin has approached you with a desire to begin an exercise program, because his physician informed him that aerobic exercise will elicit an average reduction of 10 mmHg for both systolic and diastolic blood pressures. Collin's resting blood pressure is routinely under the 200/110 mmHg level that would contraindicate exercise, and it has never approached a dangerous exaggerated pressor response of 250/115 mmHg during exercise.

Exercise prescription for hypertensive patients follows the general guidelines for the healthy population as summarized in table 2.1. Some considerations must be made based on medications and to avoid hypertensive responses to the exercise itself. Your exercise prescription for Collin, following the FITT principle and ACSM guidelines (ACSM, 2006), is as follows:

Frequency: You recommend three to seven days per week to maximize the benefits of blood pressure reduction from exercise.

Intensity: You decide on an intensity of 40 to 70% of $\dot{V}O_2R$. Collin's beta-blocker will attenuate his heart rate by about 30 beats per minute. Therefore, prescribing exercise by target heart rate, especially using methods that estimate the maximal heart rate, may not be appropriate. If stress test data on Collin had been obtained while he was taking his medication, you could use that information to determine a target HR or work rate. In Collin's case, this information is not available. Thus, you initially prescribe his intensity at a low level using 11 to 13 on the RPE scale.

Time: You decide on 30 to 60 minutes per exercise session.

Type: You recommend large muscle activities for aerobic exercise, such as walking, cycling, or swimming. You may prescribe resistance training later on, preferably using circuit weight training with high repetitions (10 to 15) and low resistance. You instruct Collin to avoid the Valsalva maneuver during his resistance exercise.

PREGNANCY

Exercise during pregnancy provides many benefits to the woman while entailing few risks to the developing fetus. Benefits to the woman include the same fitness and health benefits available to nonpregnant exercisers. In addition, women who exercise during pregnancy can generally expect a less difficult delivery and a faster return to prepregnancy weight and fitness than nonexercising pregnant women.

Women who exercise during their pregnancies report no increases in adverse effects, such as spontaneous abortions or birth abnormalities, compared with women who are sedentary during pregnancy. However, the American College of Obstetricians and Gynecologists (ACOG) has established contraindications for exercise during pregnancy (ACSM, 2006; ACOG, 2003). Women who were sedentary before their pregnancy should obtain a physician's clearance before starting an exercise program. These women should begin with light intensity, such as an RPE of 11 on the 6 to 20 scale or 20 to 39% of their HRR. Women who have been exercising regularly may continue to participate in their current exercise program, modifying the intensity, duration, and frequency as needed as the pregnancy progresses.

Exercising in extremely hot conditions during the first trimester should be avoided, because this may interfere with the closure of the neural tube, resulting in spina bifida. Moreover, exercise following the first trimester should be avoided in the supine position because mild obstruction of venous return attenuates cardiac output and may result in orthostatic hypotension. Women who have multiple gestations may need to be especially cautious not to exercise in the supine position. Scuba diving should be avoided throughout pregnancy because the fetus may be at increased risk for decompression sickness.

During the third trimester, the exercise program may need to be modified again to include exercise modalities that are weight supportive. Also, during this time, there may be a greater degree of competition between the mother and fetus for nutrients, especially glucose, which could increase the risk for maternal hypoglycemia during strenuous exercise. Pregnancy requires an additional 300 kcal per day to maintain metabolic homeostasis. Therefore, ingesting additional calories above those 300 will be needed to meet the needs of exercise.

Maximal exercise testing is generally not necessary, although submaximal testing can be performed with an end point no greater than 75% of the HRR. However, there is little point in trying to estimate aerobic fitness during pregnancy, because maximal HR declines, making such estimates inaccurate. Guidelines for an exercise prescription vary depending on the woman's exercise history. Generally, in the absence of medical or obstetric complications, exercising for 30 to 40 minutes, three to seven days per week, at an RPE between 11 and 13 is recommended. Women who have been resistance training prior to pregnancy may continue, provided there are no medical or obstetric complications. Inexperienced or novice lifters should focus the majority of their exercise routines on aerobic activities during pregnancy.

CASE STUDY 10.4
Pregnant Client

Kerri is 35 years old and has recently discovered she is pregnant. She is in her first trimester and wants to continue her exercise program. She is referred to you by her physician with permission to continue her current exercise program, provided she reduce her exercise as overall discomfort or specific symptoms dictate. Her current exercise program consists of aerobic and resistance training: She runs three or four times each week for a total of about 12 to 15 miles, and she exercises all her major muscle groups with resistance training twice a week.

Because Kerri has a very active history of exercise before her pregnancy, she should be able to adjust comfortably to an exercise program during her pregnancy. You recommend the following exercise program following ACSM and ACOG guidelines (ACSM, 2006):

Frequency: Kerri can continue exercising at least three times per week as with her regular exercise routine.

Intensity: Standard guidelines for intensity apply to pregnant women. However, because maximal HR decreases and resting HR increases during pregnancy, target HR calculations are not applicable. Furthermore, although maximal exercise testing during pregnancy has not been reported to have adverse effects, it generally is not recommended and is of limited use. Therefore, you recommend that Kerri use ratings of perceived exertion to monitor intensity. A special concern is that she avoid overheating during exercise, especially during the first trimester, when the fetus is most susceptible to heat-induced defects in development. Therefore, you instruct Kerri not to exercise in hot conditions and to remain properly hydrated.

Time: The duration of the exercise session may require daily adjustments. She should not continue an exercise session to the point of fatigue or exhaustion.

(continued)

Case Study 10.4 *(continued)*

Type: Kerri may perform weight-bearing aerobic exercise; but you point out that non-weight-bearing exercises such as stationary cycling and swimming will minimize the risk of injury, and she can perform them more comfortably—which will facilitate her continuing the exercises in the latter stages of her pregnancy. After the first trimester, she should avoid exercising in the supine position (especially if the exercise is prolonged), because it may result in a reduction in blood flow to the uterus and hypotension. She should be able to fully resume her prepregnancy exercise routines four to six weeks postpartum.

Exercise recommendations during pregnancy for women who do not exercise regularly are similar to those listed in this section. However, such women may require supervision and should be taught the signs and symptoms that indicate that they should discontinue exercise (ACSM, 2006).

CHILDREN

Since the advent of television, childhood physical activity levels have been on the decline—a trend that has increased with the widespread use of the computer as an entertainment medium. Childhood obesity is becoming epidemic, along with obesity-related diseases such as type 2 diabetes. Survey data suggest that only about 50 percent of Americans aged 12 to 21 are vigorously active on a regular basis. Exercise guidelines for children need to emphasize *the enjoyment of physical activity as a lifelong pursuit.* Regular exercise in children can reduce body fat, slow atherosclerosis and osteoporosis, and lower their chances of developing hypertension. This section provides information regarding exercise recommendations for healthy children ranging in age from 6 to 17 years, encompassing both preadolescence and adolescence.

Resistance training is appropriate for children, with only a few cautions relative to the guidelines for adults. The ACSM recommends that children not attempt maximal lifts until they reach adolescence (ACSM, 2006). Research has indicated that children can increase strength by resistance training, and, if properly supervised, such training is safe with injury risk comparable to that of adults (Burnhardt et al., 2001; Payne et al., 1997). Following resistance training, gains in muscular strength prior to puberty are mostly a result of neurological adaptations, whereas increases in strength postpuberty are likely a consequence of hypertrophy caused by higher concentrations of anabolic hormones that are present during this period.

There has been some concern regarding the potential injury to epiphyseal plates of the long bones as a result of testing or training of pre- and postpubescent children with heavy weights (e.g., 80 to 90% of the 1RM). For this reason, heavy lifting should be discouraged even though little evidence exists to prove that 1RM testing in children, if properly supervised, is harmful.

The current ACSM recommendation for resistance training in children is similar to that for older adults: high repetitions (between 8 and 15) two days per week, targeting 8 to 10 different exercises. In all other aspects, the ACSM guidelines for children's resistance training are as previously presented for adults in table 2.1. A qualified adult should always supervise children during resistance training. Be certain that you teach children (as well as all novice lifters) proper lifting technique. Remember that even large and strong children may still be physiologically immature.

Maximal aerobic testing on children is done quite routinely in pediatric testing labs to rule out cardiac problems that may be associated with chest pain, shortness of breath, and syncope, which are often reported during physical activity. Children can be tested on either an electronically braked cycle or standard treadmill; however, the treadmill seems to be the most reproducible and appropriate mode, especially when testing very young children. Adjustments to the treadmill speed and grade may be necessary to account for differences in stature and fitness levels. For more detailed information on exercise testing in children, see the ACSM *Guidelines*.

When prescribing aerobic exercise for children, activities that have a high anaerobic component are the most appropriate because they are most likely to maintain and challenge the child. Long-duration, repetitive aerobic activities usually result in early boredom and loss of interest. Estimating target heart rate using 220 − age is inappropriate for children younger than 16 years, because of a wide range of interindividual variability, and because maximal heart rate at exhaustion in a progressive test remains stable for boys and girls during the growing years and does not begin to decline until about age 16.

The principal recommendation of the ACSM (as well as the Centers for Disease Control and the U.S. Surgeon General) is that all individuals aged six years and older should engage in at least 30 minutes of moderate physical activity on most, and preferably all, days of the week (Pate et al., 1995; U.S. Department of Health and Human Services, 1996). Thus, even very young children should be engaging in regular physical activity. Preadolescents should focus on physically active play rather than on intense, structured, aerobic conditioning. Older children can benefit from vigorous aerobic training by following standard prescription guidelines, although the use of heart rate prescriptions is generally not necessary. Intensity is not as important as establishing a daily routine of activity. All children can exercise at a variety of intensities and durations; if given the choice, however, most prefer short-term intermittent activities that have a high recreational component. Most children prefer skill-related sports such as tennis, soccer, and basketball to running on a treadmill, and they generally choose outdoor bicycling rather than stationary cycling. Furthermore, children seem to tolerate activities that are repeated and have a short duration with rest periods. The least physiologically tolerable types of activities are ones that are highly anaerobic and last from 10 to 90 seconds, such as running sprints in a fitness class.

Aerobic exercise prescription for all children should focus on keeping the children active, rather than increasing their functional capacity or $\dot{V}O_2$max. Regular aerobic exercise programs that exercise children at heart rates of 170 to 180 bpm have only reported about a 10% increase in functional capacity, compared to programs for adults, which report higher increases of 15 to 30% (ACSM, 2006). Recommended activities are those that require moving the whole body, such as running, swimming, and cycling. Furthermore, because children are involved in a variety of activities throughout the day, it's best if they set aside a specific time for sustained aerobic activities. All these approaches can help maximize the volume of energy expended, which is extremely beneficial in obese children.

One concern about children's aerobic exercise is that their metabolic rate *per unit of body mass* is higher than that of adults at a given submaximal walking or running speed. Children therefore produce excessive body heat when exercising and have a higher energy expenditure than adults. Yet their immature cardiovascular systems, with low blood flow capacity in the skin, result in reduced capacity for sweating. These factors, combined with a large surface-area-to-body-mass ratio in children, result in a low tolerance to hot weather and a greater susceptibility to heat stress, especially during continuous activities. The high surface-area-to-body-mass ratio also accelerates heat loss during exposure to the cold and can increase the risk of hypothermia. Children need about 10 to 14 days to acclimate to a hot environment. They should wear loose, lightweight clothing that readily permits air flow, to allow for the evaporation of sweat. When air temperature and humidity levels are high, children should reduce activities that last longer than 30 minutes, and they should be instructed to drink 100 to 150 ml of fluid every 15 to 30 minutes, whether or not they feel thirsty. Cold water is more easily absorbed than warm water; if a sports drink is consumed instead of water, it should contain no more than 25 g of sugar per liter (Bar-Or, 1983).

Activities that involve repeated mechanical stress over a long period of time can cause overuse injuries in children. For example, excessive endurance activities can damage epiphyseal growth plates and growth tissues. For these reasons, young runners may be more prone to musculoskeletal problems than adults. Other risks include any sudden change (more than 10% in a week) in the intensity, duration, or frequency of the exercise; musculotendinous imbalances; incorrect biomechanics; and improper footwear or running surfaces.

CASE STUDY 10.5

High School Football Player

Billy is a 15-year-old high school sophomore who wants to try out for the football team next fall. He weighs 150 lb and is 5'10" tall. His coach has recommended that he increase his body weight and participate in a resistance training program over the summer to increase his strength and size.

Billy has decided to lift weights at the neighborhood YMCA, where a combination of free weights and circuit training machines are available. Because Billy has never been involved in a structured

(continued)

Case Study 10.5   *(continued)*

weightlifting program, you decide to have him begin with the circuit weight machines, exercising all his major muscle groups two times per week on Monday and Thursday. You design the following program for Billy, using a series of weightlifting machines:

Frequency: Twice per week.

Intensity: Weight loads that allow 8 to 12 repetitions.

Time: Perform one or two sets of 8 to 10 different exercises using the machines. Rest for at least one minute between sets and exercises.

Type: Progress along the circuit, training all major muscle groups, beginning with large muscle groups and ending with smaller ones. (Refer to chapter 6 for a complete description of exercises.)

In addition, you encourage Billy to participate in moderate-intensity aerobic activities for 30 minutes, three times a week. You instruct him not to engage in strenuous or prolonged aerobic conditioning, so that the extra caloric expenditure does not interfere with his desire to gain weight. You also work with him to develop an appropriate nutritional program comprising sufficient total calories as well as quality protein sources.

REFERENCES

ACSM. 2006. *ACSM's Guidelines for Exercise Testing and Prescription,* 7th ed., 205-245 Philadelphia: Lippincott Williams & Wilkins.

American College of Obstetricians and Gynecologists. 2003. Exercise during pregnancy and the postpartum period. *Clinical Obstetrics and Gynecology* 46: 496-499.

Bar-Or, O. 1983. *Pediatric Sports Medicine for the Practitioner: From Physiologic Principles to Clinical Applications.* New York: Springer.

Bernhardt, D.T., J. Gomez, M.D. Johnson, et al. 2001. Strength training by children and adolescents. *Pediatrics* 107: 1470-1472.

Fagard R. 2001. Exercise characteristics and the blood pressure response to dynamic physical training. *Medicine and Science in Sports and Exercise* 33: S484-S492.

Pate, R.R., M. Pratt, S.N. Blair, W.L. Haskell, C.A. Macera, C. Bouchard, D. Buchner, W. Ettinger, G.W. Heath, and A.C. King.1995. Physical activity and public health. A recommendation from the Centers for Disease Control and Prevention and the American College of Sports Medicine. *Journal of the American Medical Association* 273: 402-407.

Payne, V.G., J.R. Morrow, L. Johnson, and S.N. Dalton. 1997. Resistance training in children and youth: A meta-analysis. *Research Quarterly for Exercise and Sport* 68: 80-88.

U.S. Department of Health and Human Services. 1996. *Physical Activity and Health: A Report of the Surgeon General.* Atlanta, GA: U.S. Department of Health and Human Services, Centers for Disease Control and Prevention, National Center for Chronic Disease Prevention and Health Promotion.

Appendix

ADDITIONAL CASE STUDIES WITH MULTIPLE-CHOICE QUESTIONS

CASE STUDY A.1
Young Adult Client

Marina is a 36-year-old nonsmoker who weighs 108 lb (49 kg) and is 5'1" (155 cm) tall. She lifts weights and jogs several times per week. Her father had a heart attack when he was 49 years old, and her mother was diagnosed with breast cancer when she was 58 years old. Marina has recently had a complete fitness evaluation, which revealed the following: Her resting blood pressure and heart rate are 98/64 mmHg and 68 bpm, respectively. Her lipid profile is as follows: total cholesterol of 182 mg · dl^{-1}, LDL cholesterol of 118 mg · dl^{-1}, HDL cholesterol of 52 mg · dl^{-1}. Fasting glucose is 93 mg · dl^{-1}. Her estimated $\dot{V}O_2$max is 42 ml · min^{-1} · kg^{-1} (80th percentile). Other fitness measures are 1RM bench press 85 lb, or 38.5 kg (90th percentile), 25 partial curl-ups ("excellent"), and 31 cm sit-and-reach score on box with 26 cm at foot line ("fair").

1. Marina's body mass index is
   a. in the "underweight" category
   b. 20.4 kg · m^{-2}
   c. 24.6 kg · m^{-2}
   d. 29.0 kg · m^{-2}

2. Which of the following ACSM risk factors does Marina have?
   a. obesity
   b. family history
   c. hypercholesterolemia
   d. negative risk factor for high HDL

3. To which risk stratification category does Marina belong?

    a. low-risk

    b. moderate-risk

    c. high-risk

4. If Marina wishes to exercise in your facility, will she need physician clearance first?

    a. yes, if the exercise is to be vigorous; but no, if moderate

    b. yes, if the exercise is to be moderate or vigorous

    c. no, for moderate or vigorous exercise

5. What would be Marina's target heart rate at 70% of $\dot{V}O_2R$, using the %HRmax method? (Hint: See table 3.1.)

    a. 129 bpm

    b. 155 bpm

    c. 172 bpm

    d. 184 bpm

6. What would be Marina's target heart rate at 70% of $\dot{V}O_2R$, using the %HRR method?

    a. 81 bpm

    b. 116 bpm

    c. 136 bpm

    d. 149 bpm

7. What would be Marina's gross oxygen consumption at 70% of $\dot{V}O_2R$?

    a. 38.5 ml $\cdot$ min^{-1} $\cdot$ kg^{-1}

    b. 30.5 ml $\cdot$ min^{-1} $\cdot$ kg^{-1}

    c. 29.4 ml $\cdot$ min^{-1} $\cdot$ kg^{-1}

    d. 27.0 ml $\cdot$ min^{-1} $\cdot$ kg^{-1}

8. For indoor aerobic exercise, Marina would like to walk on a treadmill. If she walks at 3.5 mph, what % grade would allow her to exercise at 70% of $\dot{V}O_2R$?

    a. 8%

    b. 9%

    c. 10%

    d. She cannot walk at 3.5 mph and attain the desired $\dot{V}O_2$ on a treadmill.

9. What would be Marina's net caloric expenditure at 70% of $\dot{V}O_2R$?

   a. 6.6 kcal $\cdot$ min^{-1}

   b. 7.5 kcal $\cdot$ min^{-1}

   c. 9.5 kcal $\cdot$ min^{-1}

   d. 10.3 kcal $\cdot$ min^{-1}

10. Based on Marina's fitness assessment, which component of fitness should she most work to improve?

    a. body composition

    b. aerobic capacity

    c. muscular strength

    d. flexibility

CASE STUDY A.2
Young Adult Client

Heather is 43 years old, weighs 142 lb (64.5 kg), and is 5'5" (165 cm) tall. She is a former one-pack-a-day cigarette smoker, having quit smoking two years ago. She has a sedentary job but sometimes takes a 15-minute walk at lunch time. Her father had coronary angioplasty when he was 61 years old. Her resting blood pressure and heart rate are 132/84 mmHg and 78 bpm, respectively. Her lipid profile is total cholesterol of 194 mg $\cdot$ dl^{-1}, LDL of 134 mg $\cdot$ dl^{-1}, and HDL of 45 mg $\cdot$ dl^{-1}. Fasting glucose is 102 mg $\cdot$ dl^{-1}. Her estimated $\dot{V}O_2$max is 27 ml $\cdot$ min$^{1}\cdot$ kg^{-1} (10th percentile). Other fitness measures are an estimated body fat (skinfolds) of 28% (40th percentile), 12 modified push-ups (nearly "good"), 14 partial curl-ups (nearly "good"), and 24 cm sit-and-reach score on box with 26 cm at foot line ("needs improvement").

11. Which of the following ACSM risk factors does Heather have?

    a. obesity

    b. family history

    c. sedentary lifestyle

    d. hypercholesterolemia

    e. impaired fasting glucose

    f. c, d, and e

12. To which risk stratification category does Heather belong?
    a. low-risk
    b. moderate-risk
    c. high-risk

13. If Heather wishes to exercise in your facility, will she need physician clearance first?
    a. yes, if the exercise is to be vigorous; but no, if moderate
    b. yes, if the exercise is to be moderate or vigorous
    c. no, for moderate or vigorous exercise

14. What would be Heather's target heart rate at 50% of $\dot{V}O_2R$, using the %HRR method?
    a. 177 bpm
    b. 128 bpm
    c. 99 bpm
    d. 89 bpm

15. What would be Heather's target workload on a leg cycle ergometer at 50% of $\dot{V}O_2R$?
    a. 50 W
    b. 125 W
    c. 450 kg · m · min^{-1}
    d. 600 kg · m · min^{-1}

16. If Heather is cycling on a Monark bike ergometer at 50 rpm, what resistance setting in kg would place her at 50% of $\dot{V}O_2R$?
    a. 0.5 kg
    b. 1.0 kg
    c. 1.5 kg
    d. 2.0 kg

17. For improving cardiorespiratory fitness, what frequency of exercise should you recommend for Heather?
    a. two or three times per week
    b. three to five times per week
    c. four to six times per week
    d. five to seven times per week

18. For improving muscular strength and muscular endurance, what repetition range for resistance exercise should you recommend for Heather?

    a. 4-6

    b. 6-10

    c. 8-12

    d. 10-15

19. For improving muscular fitness, what frequency of exercise should you recommend for Heather?

    a. two or three times per week

    b. three to five times per week

    c. four to six times per week

    d. five to seven times per week

20. When she performs flexibility exercises, which of the following would be contraindicated for Heather?

    a. bouncing to achieve a greater stretch

    b. curving the upper body forward while performing a hamstring stretch

    c. performing a "hurdler's" stretch with the opposite knee bent rearward

    d. all of the above

CASE STUDY A.3

Weight Loss Client

Frank is 27 years old, weighs 212 lb (96.4 kg), and is 5'8" (173 cm) tall. He is a sedentary nonsmoker. His father was diagnosed with type 2 diabetes at 51 years of age, and his mother had a heart attack when she was 62. His resting blood pressure and heart rate are 146/94 mmHg and 84 bpm, respectively. His lipid profile is total cholesterol of 234 mg · dl^{-1}, LDL of 142 mg · dl^{-1}, and HDL of 46 mg · dl^{-1}. Fasting glucose is 106 mg · dl^{-1}. After complaining of chest pain during a softball game, he was given a stress test. His measured $\dot{V}O_2$max was 24 ml · min^{-1} · kg^{-1} (<10th percentile). His maximal heart rate was 198 bpm. There were no signs or symptoms of heart disease, and his physician has cleared him for exercise. His body fat has been measured by hydrostatic weighing as 35% (<10th percentile).

21. In what category is Frank's body mass index?
    a. class II obesity
    b. class I obesity
    c. overweight
    d. normal

22. How many ACSM risk factors does Frank have?
    a. four
    b. five
    c. six
    d. seven

23. What is Frank's current lean body weight?
    a. 74 lb (33.6 kg)
    b. 118 lb (53.6 kg)
    c. 127 lb (57.7 kg)
    d. 138 lb (62.7 kg)

24. What would Frank weigh at 20% body fat, assuming no change in his lean body mass?
    a. 158 lb (71.7 kg)
    b. 172 lb (78.2 kg)
    c. 180 lb (81.8 kg)
    d. 197 lb (89.5 kg)

25. How long should Frank take to reach his goal weight at 20% body fat?
    a. 20 to 40 weeks
    b. 6 months to a year
    c. 1 to 2 years
    d. 15 to 30 weeks

26. What would be Frank's target heart rate at 50% of $\dot{V}O_2R$, using the %HRR method?
    a. 139 bpm
    b. 141 bpm
    c. 151 bpm
    d. 163 bpm

27. What walking speed on flat ground would place Frank at 50% of $\dot{V}O_2R$?

    a. 2.5 mph (4.0 kph)

    b. 2.8 mph (4.5 kph)

    c. 3.4 mph (5.5 kph)

    d. 3.8 mph (6.1 kph)

28. What work rate on a leg cycle ergometer would place Frank at 50% of $\dot{V}O_2R$?

    a. 100 W

    b. 75 W

    c. 400 kg·m·min^{-1}

    d. 360 kg·m·min^{-1}

29. What would be Frank's net caloric expenditure at 50% of $\dot{V}O_2R$?

    a. 5.0 kcal·min^{-1}

    b. 6.6 kcal·min^{-1}

    c. 7.5 kcal·min^{-1}

    d. 9.5 kcal·min^{-1}

30. If Frank walks every day, how many minutes per day would be required for him to lose 0.5 lb (0.23 kg) of fat each week through the exercise alone?

    a. 38 minutes

    b. 45 minutes

    c. 50 minutes

    d. 60 minutes

CASE STUDY A.4
Older Adult Client

Roberto is 71 years old, weighs 176 lb (80 kg), and is 5' 10" (178 cm) tall. He is a pipe smoker. He likes to play golf, but he uses a cart. His sister had bypass surgery when she was 64 years old. His resting blood pressure and heart rate are 128/82 mmHg and

(continued)

90 bpm, respectively. His lipid profile is total cholesterol of 204 mg · dl⁻¹, LDL of 126 mg · dl⁻¹, and HDL of 39 mg · dl⁻¹. Fasting glucose is 94 mg · dl⁻¹. His estimated $\dot{V}O_2$max is 18 ml · min⁻¹ · kg⁻¹ (<10th percentile). Other fitness measures are six push-ups ("fair"), nine partial curl-ups ("fair"), and 19 cm sit-and-reach score on box with 26 cm at foot line ("fair"). He has moderate to severe arthritis in his knees.

31. Which of the following ACSM risk factors does Roberto have?

    a. family history

    b. sedentary lifestyle

    c. obesity

    d. dyslipidemia

    e. a, b, and d

    f. all of the above

32. To which risk stratification category does Roberto belong?

    a. low-risk

    b. moderate-risk

    c. high-risk

33. To improve his muscular strength and muscular endurance, how many different resistance training exercises should Roberto perform?

    a. 3 or 4

    b. 5 or 6

    c. 6 to 8

    d. 8 to 10

34. To improve his muscular strength and muscular endurance, what repetition range should Roberto perform *according to the ACSM?*

    a. 6 to 8

    b. 8 to 12

    c. 10 to 15

    d. 12 to 15

35. For which of the following reasons is a target heart rate likely to be inaccurate in Roberto's case?

   a. The elderly do not have a linear response of heart rate to workload.

   b. In the elderly, %HRR and %$\dot{V}O_2R$ are not closely related.

   c. You don't know Roberto's true maximum HR.

   d. Arthritis affects the HR response to exercise.

36. If you were to prescribe Roberto a target HR, what would it be at 40% of $\dot{V}O_2R$ using the %HRmax method? (Hint: See table 3.1.)

   a. 95 bpm

   b. 114 bpm

   c. 122 bpm

   d. 141 bpm

37. If you were to prescribe Roberto a target HR, what would it be at 40% of $\dot{V}O_2R$ using the %HRR method?

   a. 95 bpm

   b. 114 bpm

   c. 122 bpm

   d. 141 bpm

38. Which mode of cardiorespiratory exercise would be preferred for Roberto?

   a. jogging

   b. bench stepping

   c. water aerobics

   d. a or b

39. What workload on an arm ergometer would place Roberto at 40% of $\dot{V}O_2R$?

   a. 26 W

   b. 32 W

   c. 250 kg · m · min^{-1}

   d. 360 kg · m · min^{-1}

40. What RPE range would approximate 40 to 60% of $\dot{V}O_2R$ for Roberto?

    a. 12 to 14

    b. 13 to 15

    c. 14 to 16

    d. 15 to 17

CASE STUDY A.5

Client With Myocardial Infarction

Akim is a sedentary 45-year-old smoker who weighs 245 lb (111.4 kg) and is 5'10" (178 cm) tall. He was recently admitted to the hospital complaining of chest pain. His cardiac blood enzymes were elevated along with his ST segments, confirming a myocardial infarction in progress. Akim was rushed to the catheterization lab where it was determined that his left anterior descending artery was blocked at the proximal end. He underwent percutaneous transluminal coronary angioplasty (PTCA), which was successful. His ejection fraction is 55%. Two weeks have passed, and Andy is ready to begin your phase II cardiac rehabilitation program. A recent nonmaximal stress test following the Bruce protocol was terminated at 85% of the predicted maximal heart rate and revealed the following data:

Resting HR: 80 bpm

Resting BP: 142/90 mmHg

Peak HR: 145 bpm (test terminated at ~85% of age-estimated HRmax)

Peak BP: 182/96 mmHg

Test terminated at 8:00 minutes into Bruce protocol (3.4 mph, 14% grade)

Medications: Aspirin, Cardizem

Other information from Akim's chart indicated a lipid profile with a total cholesterol of 250 mg · dl^{-1}, LDL of 160 mg · dl^{-1}, and HDL of 35 mg · dl^{-1}. His father died of a heart attack at age 56. Andy is currently working as a salesman for a large paper company and has no physically active recreational pursuits.

41. How many risk factors does Akim have for coronary artery disease?

    a. two
    b. three
    c. four
    d. five

42. What is Akim's body mass index?

    a. 30.3 kg · m^{-2}
    b. 35.1 kg · m^{-2}
    c. 42.6 kg · m^{-2}

43. In which ACSM risk stratification category does Akim belong?

    a. low-risk
    b. moderate-risk
    c. high-risk

44. Based on the previous stress test information, at approximately what gross oxygen consumption was the stress test stopped?

    a. 30.7 ml · min^{-1} · kg^{-1}
    b. 35.5 ml · min^{-1} · kg^{-1}
    c. 42.9 ml · min^{-1} · kg^{-1}
    d. 54.0 ml · min^{-1} · kg^{-1}

45. Approximately how many kilocalories per minute (gross) was Akim expending during the final stage of his treadmill test?

    a. 10
    b. 15
    c. 20
    d. 25

46. Calculate a target heart rate for Akim at 60% and 80% of $\dot{V}O_2R$, using the %HRR method.

    a. 140 to 182 bpm
    b. 137 to 156 bpm
    c. 155 to 183 bpm
    d. 142 to 156 bpm

47. What would be Akim's target heart rate at 70% of $\dot{V}O_2R$ using the %HRmax method? (Hint: See table 3.1.)

    a. 120 bpm

    b. 135 bpm

    c. 147 bpm

    d. 169 bpm

48. You want to prescribe Akim a weight training program when he completes phase II of the rehabilitation program. Based on the ACSM guidelines, what should the frequency and intensity be?

    a. two or three days per week, 10- to 15-rep range

    b. five or six days per week, 80% of the 1RM

    c. seven days per week as tolerated

    d. two days per week, light weight and very high reps (>15)

49. Traditionally, Akim's phase II rehabilitation is expected to last for how long?

    a. 6 weeks

    b. 8 weeks

    c. 12 weeks

    d. 24 months

50. At the conclusion of Akim's phase II program, you want to reevaluate his aerobic fitness. Which of the following tests can you perform without the presence of a physician?

    a. submaximal

    b. maximal

    c. either submaximal or maximal

    d. neither submaximal nor maximal

CASE STUDY A.6

Client With Pacemaker

Li is a 50-year-old sedentary male who was seen by his physician with the primary complaint of tiredness. His weight and height are 170 lb (77.3 kg) and 5'9" (175 cm). He is a nonsmoker with no history of heart disease in his family. A blood lipid profile reported a total cholesterol level of 189 mg·dl⁻¹, HDL of 36 mg·dl⁻¹, and LDL of 135 mg·dl⁻¹. A resting ECG determined a bradycardic heart rate. Li was referred to a cardiologist who specialized in the electrophysiology of the heart. He diagnosed chronotropic incompetence, with adequate sinus node function and high-grade AV block. Therefore, it was recommended that Li receive a DDD pacemaker so that AV synchrony, rate responsiveness, and atrial tracking would occur during activity. Three weeks following the implantation of the pacemaker, he underwent a maximal exercise test before entering your phase II cardiac rehabilitation program, and his estimated $\dot{V}O_2$max was 35 ml·min⁻¹·kg⁻¹. His resting heart rate and blood pressure were 70 bpm and 110/70 mmHg. Peak heart rate and blood pressure were 160 bpm and 172/80 mmHg, respectively.

51. How many coronary artery disease risk factors (do not include his pacemaker) does Li have?

    a. one
    b. two
    c. three
    d. four

52. What is Li's body mass index?

    a. 20 kg·m⁻²
    b. 25 kg·m⁻²
    c. 30 kg·m⁻²
    d. 42 kg·m⁻²

53. Based on Li's BMI, what classification of disease risk is he in?

    a. underweight
    b. normal
    c. overweight
    d. obese

54. What would be Li's target heart rate at 70% of $\dot{V}O_2$R using the %HRR method?

    a. 119 bpm
    b. 133 bpm
    c. 140 bpm
    d. 148 bpm

55. To reach his target HR, Li must walk 3.0 mph at a grade of 10%. What is his estimated gross $\dot{V}O_2$ at this speed and grade?

    a. 15 ml $\cdot$ min^{-1} $\cdot$ kg^{-1}

    b. 20 ml $\cdot$ min^{-1} $\cdot$ kg^{-1}

    c. 26 ml $\cdot$ min^{-1} $\cdot$ kg^{-1}

    d. 29 ml $\cdot$ min^{-1} $\cdot$ kg^{-1}

56. How many gross kcal per minute would Li be expending at his peak $\dot{V}O_2$?

    a. 13.5

    b. 15

    c. 23

    d. There is not enough information to calculate his caloric expenditure.

57. To exercise at 60% of $\dot{V}O_2R$ on an 8-inch-high (20.3 cm) bench, what stepping rate would he need to use?

    a. 15 steps $\cdot$ min^{-1}

    b. 28 steps $\cdot$ min^{-1}

    c. 30 steps $\cdot$ min^{-1}

    d. 42 steps $\cdot$ min^{-1}

58. Li has expressed an interest in using a stationary bicycle. What work rate should you set to achieve 70% of $\dot{V}O_2R$?

    a. 100 W

    b. 130 W

    c. 150 W

    d. 200 W

59. Li wants to begin a very light resistance training program and also perform range-of-motion exercises to strengthen his upper body. When should he be able to begin?

    a. immediately after implantation

    b. one week after implantation

    c. two to three weeks after implantation

    d. one month after implantation

60. How often should Li's resistance training and range-of-motion exercises be performed?

    a. one day per week

    b. two or three days per week

    c. four days per week

    d. Resistance training and range-of-motion exercises should not be performed during the same week.

CASE STUDY A.7

Client With Type 1 Diabetes

Alejandro is a 32-year-old who was diagnosed with type 1 diabetes at the age of 10. His treatment consists of twice-daily injections of both short-acting and intermediate-acting insulin. He weighs 143 lb (65 kg) and is 5' 7" (170 cm) tall. His most recent fasting blood test results were total cholesterol of 221 mg · dl^{-1}, LDL of 140 mg · dl^{-1}, and HDL of 42 mg · dl^{-1}. Fasting glucose was 123 mg · dl^{-1}. His resting blood pressure and heart rate are 124/82 mmHg and 76 bpm, respectively. He has recently tried jogging to "get in better shape" but has experienced several bouts of hypoglycemia. He visited his physician, who has referred him to you for a fitness evaluation and exercise prescription. Results of his fitness evaluation include an estimated $\dot{V}O_2$max of 39 ml · min^{-1} · kg^{-1} (30th percentile), an estimated body fat (skinfolds) of 20% (40th percentile), 22 push-ups (approximately "good"), 18 partial curl-ups (approximately "good"), and 18 cm sit-and-reach score on box with 26 cm at foot line ("needs improvement").

61. To which ACSM risk category does Alejandro belong?

    a. low-risk

    b. moderate-risk

    c. high-risk

62. What should be Alejandro's first step in adjusting his routine to avoid exercise-induced hypoglycemia?

    a. Increase insulin dosage before exercise.

    b. Decrease insulin dosage before exercise.

    c. Consume extra carbohydrate throughout the day.

    d. Reduce carbohydrate consumption before exercise.

63. At what frequency should Alejandro begin his aerobic training program?

    a. twice per week

    b. three times per week

    c. five times per week

    d. every day

64. At what duration should Alejandro begin his aerobic training program?

    a. 10 to 20 minutes

    b. 20 to 30 minutes

    c. 30 to 40 minutes

    d. 50 to 60 minutes

65. Which of the following workloads would place Alejandro at 60% of $\dot{V}O_2R$?

    a. jogging at 9.7 mph

    b. walking at 3 mph up a 4% grade

    c. stationary biking at 150 W

    d. stepping 26 times per minute on a 10-inch (25.4 cm) bench

66. What would be Alejandro's target HR at 60% of $\dot{V}O_2R$ using the %HRR method?

    a. 113 bpm

    b. 123 bpm

    c. 133 bpm

    d. 143 bpm

67. Alejandro measures his blood glucose a few minutes before a planned exercise session and records a value of 85 mg · dl^{-1}. What should he do?

    a. Remeasure it, because that can't be correct.

    b. Cancel the exercise session.

    c. Eat 20 to 30 g of carbohydrate, remeasure after 15 minutes, and exercise if it is then above 100 mg · dl^{-1}.

    d. Begin exercise.

68. Alejandro measures his blood glucose a few minutes before a planned exercise session and records a value of 260 mg · dl^{-1}. What should he do?

    a. Begin exercise.

    b. Cancel exercise.

    c. Eat 20 to 30 g of carbohydrate and then exercise.

    d. Check for urinary ketones; if present, cancel exercise.

69. During an exercise session, Alejandro experiences weakness and light-headedness. What should he do?

    a. Call 911.

    b. Eat a fast-acting source of sugar to relieve the symptoms.

    c. Lie down and rest until the symptoms go away.

    d. Continue exercising until the symptoms go away.

70. At what repetition range should Alejandro perform resistance training?

    a. 8 to 12

    b. 10 to 15

    c. 15 to 20

    d. He should not do resistance training.

CASE STUDY A.8
Client With Type 2 Diabetes

William is 62 years old and was diagnosed with type 2 diabetes last month. He has been placed on oral hypoglycemic therapy, has seen a nutritionist about improving his diet, and has now been referred to you for an exercise program. A stress test showed that his $\dot{V}O_2max$ is 18 ml · min^{-1} · kg^{-1} (<10th percentile); his maximal heart rate is166 bpm. There were no signs or symptoms of heart disease. He weighs 320 lb (145.5 kg) and is 5' 11" (180.3 cm) tall. His blood test showed a total cholesterol of 284 mg · dl^{-1}, LDL of 146 mg · dl^{-1}, and HDL of 37 mg · dl^{-1}. Fasting glucose is 184 mg · dl^{-1}. His resting blood pressure and heart rate are 124/82 mmHg and 76 bpm, respectively.

71. In what category is William's body mass index?
    a. overweight
    b. class I obesity
    c. class II obesity
    d. class III obesity

72. What would be William's target weight at a BMI of 25 kg · m^{-2}?
    a. 179 lb
    b. 196 lb
    c. 218 lb
    d. 242 lb

73. What intensity range should William be initially prescribed?
    a. 40 to 60% $\dot{V}O_2R$
    b. 50 to 70% $\dot{V}O_2R$
    c. 50 to 85% $\dot{V}O_2R$
    d. 60 to 80% $\dot{V}O_2R$

74. After he has progressed through several weeks of aerobic exercise training, what frequency and duration should William be prescribed?
    a. 20 to 30 minutes, three to five times per week
    b. 20 to 30 minutes, five to seven times per week
    c. 50 to 60 minutes, three to five times per week
    d. 50 to 60 minutes, five to seven times per week

75. If you prescribed a target heart rate at 50% of $\dot{V}O_2R$, what would that be using the %HRR method?
    a. 102 bpm
    b. 117 bpm
    c. 121 bpm
    d. 132 bpm

76. What walking speed should William be able to maintain on a flat treadmill, assuming 50% of $\dot{V}O_2R$ as the target intensity?
    a. 2.1 mph (3.4 kph)
    b. 2.7 mph (4.3 kph)

c. 3.2 mph (5.1 kph)

d. 3.5 mph (5.6 kph)

77. What total duration of exercise at 50% of $\dot{V}O_2R$ would William need to accumulate to lose 1 lb (0.45 kg) of fat from the exercise alone?

    a. 4.5 hours

    b. 7.5 hours

    c. 11 hours

    d. 14 hours

78. Prior to one particular exercise session, William measures his blood glucose and records a value of 226 mg · dl^{-1}. What should he do?

    a. Begin exercise.

    b. Cancel the exercise.

    c. Wait 15 minutes and remeasure.

    d. Check for urinary ketones; if present, cancel exercise.

79. Prior to one particular exercise session, William recorded a blood glucose of 176 mg · dl^{-1}. Immediately after that exercise session he recorded a value of 124 mg · dl^{-1}. What should he do?

    a. Eat a source of fast-acting sugar.

    b. Go about his day but be aware of possible hypoglycemia.

    c. Make an immediate appointment with his physician.

    d. Drink a glass of water, wait 15 minutes, and remeasure.

80. Nine months after beginning his exercise and diet program, William has lost 52 lb (23.6 kg). He has started to experience hypoglycemia during his exercise sessions. What is the best choice for handling this new situation?

    a. Increase his consumption of total daily calories.

    b. Consume 20 to 30 g of carbohydrate before each exercise bout.

    c. Consult his physician about reducing his hypoglycemic medication.

    d. Ignore the hypoglycemia until he is at his goal weight.

CASE STUDY A.9
Client With Peripheral Arterial Disease

Miguel is a 65-year-old sedentary smoker who weighs 234 lb (106.4 kg) and is 6'3" (191 cm) tall. Lately, Miguel has noticed that when he walks, he experiences a burning, tight sensation in his calf muscles. After bringing this to his physician's attention, he was diagnosed with peripheral arterial disease (PAD). Because of a high association of cardiovascular disease and stroke in patients with PAD, Miguel's physician decided to do a treadmill test to evaluate his blood pressure and heart rate during activity. The treadmill test was prematurely stopped because of ischemic leg pain. Therefore, the physician decided to repeat the test using a stationary cycle ergometer. Miguel reached a maximal work rate of 200 W with no signs or symptoms of heart disease. His resting heart rate and blood pressure were 80 bpm and 150/90 mmHg, respectively. His peak heart rate and blood pressure were 152 bpm and 250/110 mmHg, respectively. A blood lipid profile reported a total cholesterol level of 189 mg · dl^{-1}, HDL of 40 mg · dl^{-1} and LDL of 120 mg · dl^{-1}. Miguel was prescribed a beta-blocker to treat his high blood pressure and pentoxifylline for his PAD. He was then referred to you for exercise in your phase III cardiac rehabilitation program.

81. Based on the previous information, what risk factors does Miguel have for coronary artery disease?
    a. sedentary behavior, cigarette smoking, hypertension
    b. hypercholesterolemia
    c. obesity
    d. a and b
    e. a and c

82. To which risk stratification category does Miguel belong?
    a. low-risk
    b. moderate-risk
    c. high-risk

83. What ankle-to-arm index for systolic blood pressure is typical of patients with severe PAD?
    a. 0.91 to 1.30
    b. 0.41 to 0.90
    c. <0.40

84. Which modality of exercise would be the most beneficial for improving Miguel's tolerance to leg pain?
    a. weight-bearing exercise
    b. swimming
    c. resistance training
    d. cycling

85. If Miguel stops a walking session because of leg pain, what should you do to extend his exercise session and improve his cardiovascular health?
    a. Encourage him to run.
    b. Have him seek motivational counseling.
    c. Include non-weight-bearing exercises until the leg pain subsides.
    d. Prescribe isometric leg lifts.

86. When prescribing exercise intensity for Miguel using the claudication scale, what grade should be used?
    a. 1
    b. 2
    c. 3
    d. 4

87. What is Miguel's estimated gross $\dot{V}O_2$max from his stationary cycle test?
    a. 20 ml · min^{-1} · kg^{-1}
    b. 27.3 ml · min^{-1} · kg^{-1}
    c. 30.2 ml · min^{-1} · kg^{-1}
    d. 35 ml · min^{-1} · kg^{-1}

88. Approximately how many net kilocalories per minute was Miguel expending at this work rate?
    a. 12.7
    b. 14.5
    c. 20.2
    d. 28.7

89. Based on Miguel's stationary cycle test, what would be his target work rate at 50% of $\dot{V}O_2R$?
    a. 83 W
    b. 100 W
    c. 115 W
    d. 122 W

90. What effect would the beta-blocker have on Miguel's exercise prescription?

    a. It would attenuate his target heart rate.
    b. It may decrease time to claudication.
    c. It would have no effect.
    d. a and b

CASE STUDY A.10

Pregnant Client

Gwen is a 24-year-old sedentary woman who has just learned that she is pregnant for the first time. She has heard that exercise can help her during her pregnancy and delivery, so she has come to your fitness facility to start an exercise program.

91. Which of the following is true concerning Gwen's participation in an exercise program according to ACOG/ACSM guidelines?

    a. She should obtain physician clearance before beginning.
    b. If you screen her in your facility and she meets low- or moderate-risk criteria, she can begin the program without physician clearance.
    c. At her age, she can begin right away without any screening or clearance.

92. Once Gwen has properly begun her exercise program, which weightlifting exercises should she avoid after the first trimester?

    a. flat bench press
    b. supine leg press
    c. squats
    d. a and b

93. In which trimester is it most important to have adequate hydration and to wear appropriate clothing for heat dissipation?

    a. first
    b. second
    c. third
    d. They are all equally important.

94. Which of the following statements about exercise and pregnancy is true?

    a. Healthy pregnant women do not need to limit their exercise for fear of adverse effects.

    b. Spontaneous abortion, preterm labor, and birth abnormalities are more likely in women who exercise during pregnancy.

    c. Strenuous exercise during pregnancy may result in babies with lighter birth weights.

    d. a and c

95. Maximal exercise testing during pregnancy

    a. is recommended to determine exercise intensity

    b. is rarely done and generally not recommended

    c. is commonly used to establish $\dot{V}O_2$max during pregnancy

    d. will result in sudden death to the mother

96. During pregnancy, how should aerobic exercise intensity be determined?

    a. %$\dot{V}O_2$R

    b. rating of perceived exertion

    c. %HRR

    d. %$\dot{V}O_2$max

97. Most women can return to their prepregnancy exercise routines within what time frame?

    a. zero to two weeks postpartum

    b. two to four weeks postpartum

    c. four to six weeks postpartum

    d. six to eight weeks postpartum

98. Which of the following benefits can Gwen expect from exercising during her pregnancy?

    a. easier delivery

    b. improved cardiovascular and muscular fitness

    c. more rapid return to prepregnancy weight

    d. all of the above

99. Why is prescribing exercise intensity via a target heart rate during pregnancy not recommended?
    a. There are chronotropic alterations during pregnancy that would affect the calculated value for the target heart rate.
    b. Heart rate is too irregular to monitor during pregnancy.
    c. Heart rate and $\dot{V}O_2$ are not linearly related during pregnancy.
    d. The fetal heart rate interferes with the measurement of the maternal heart rate.

100. To avoid injury during the latter stages of pregnancy, what should Gwen do?
    a. Stop all exercise during the third trimester.
    b. Never exercise above a heart rate of 140 bpm.
    c. Substitute non-weight-bearing exercises for weight-bearing exercises.
    d. Exercise only in the early morning.

ANSWERS TO QUESTIONS

Case Study A.1

1. b [Calculate BMI as lb $\times$ 703 / in^2, or kg / height in meters^2.]

2. b [Father had MI before age 55; see table 1.1.]

3. a [Young, only one risk factor; see table 1.1.]

4. c [Low-risk does not need physician clearance; see table 1.1.]

5. b [Estimate HRmax as 220 – age; multiply by factor in table 3.1.]

6. d [Target HR = (fractional intensity)(HRmax – HRrest) + HRrest.]

7. b [Target $\dot{V}O_2$ = (fractional intensity)($\dot{V}O_2$max – 3.5) + 3.5.]

8. c [Calculate speed in m · min^{-1} as mph $\times$ 26.8; solve for grade in the following equation: $\dot{V}O_2$ during walking = 3.5 + 0.1(speed) + 1.8(speed)(fractional grade).]

9.a [Net $\dot{V}O_2=$ gross $\dot{V}O_2 - 3.5$; calculate body mass in kg as lb / 2.2; convert $\dot{V}O_2$ in ml $\cdot$ min$^{-1}\cdot$ kg^{-1} to L $\cdot$ min^{-1}; multiply $\dot{V}O_2$ in L $\cdot$ min^{-1} by 5 to attain kcal $\cdot$ min^{-1}.]

10.d [Sit-and-reach score is only at 40th percentile.]

Case Study A.2

11.f [Accumulates less than 30 minutes of moderate exercise most days of the week; LDL cholesterol is >130 mg $\cdot$ dl^{-1}; fasting glucose is >100 mg $\cdot$ dl^{-1}; see table 1.1.]

12.b [Three risk factors; see table 1.1.]

13.a [Moderate-risk clients need physician clearance for vigorous, but not moderate, exercise; see table 1.1.]

14.b [Estimate HRmax as 220 – age; target HR = (fractional intensity)(HRmax – HRrest) + HRrest.]

15.a [Target $\dot{V}O_2 = $ (fractional intensity)($\dot{V}O_2$max – 3.5) + 3.5; calculate body mass in kg as lb / 2.2; solve for workload in the following equation: $\dot{V}O_2$ during leg cycling $= 7 + 1.8$(workrate) / (body mass); calculate power in W as workload in kg $\cdot$ m $\cdot$ min^{-1} divided by 6.]

16.b [Solve for resistance setting in the following equation: workload = (resistance setting)(6 m)(rpm).]

17.b [See table 2.1.]

18.c [See table 2.1.]

19.a [See table 2.1.]

20.d [Static is preferred over ballistic; spine should remain in neutral position; excessive torsion at knee.]

Case Study A.3

21.b [Calculate BMI as lb $\times$ 703 / in^2; see table 1.2.]

22.c [Obesity, sedentary behavior, maternal MI prior to 65 years of age, hypertension, LDL >130 mg $\cdot$ dl^{-1}, fasting glucose $\geq$100 mg $\cdot$ dl^{-1}; see table 1.1.]

23.d [Fat weight = (% fat)(total body weight); lean body weight = total body weight – fat weight.]

24.b [Desired weight = (current weight)(1 – current % fat) / (1 – desired % fat); i.e., desired weight = LBW / (desired % lean).]

25.a [Recommended rate of fat loss is 1 to 2 lb per week, or 0.45 to 0.9 kg]

26.b [Target HR = (fractional intensity)(HRmax – HRrest) + HRrest; *Note:* Use known HRmax.]

27.d [Target $\dot{V}O_2$ = (fractional intensity)($\dot{V}O_2$max – 3.5) + 3.5; solve for walking speed in the following equation: $\dot{V}O_2$ during walking = 3.5 + 0.1(speed) + 1.8(speed)(fractional grade). *Note:* Because the grade is zero, the last term drops out; calculate speed in mph as $m \cdot min^{-1}$ / 26.8.]

28.d [Calculate body mass in kg as lb / 2.2; solve for workload in the following equation: $\dot{V}O_2$ during leg cycling = 7 + 1.8(workrate) / (body mass).]

29.a [Net $\dot{V}O_2$ = gross $\dot{V}O_2$ – 3.5; convert $\dot{V}O_2$ in $ml \cdot min^{-1} \cdot kg^{-1}$ to $L \cdot min^{-1}$; multiply $\dot{V}O_2$ in $L \cdot min^{-1}$ by 5 to attain $kcal \cdot min^{-1}$.]

30.c [1 lb of fat contains 3,500 kcal; divide one half this value by the net caloric expenditure rate to obtain total minutes needed; divide this value by 7 for daily time required.]

Case Study A.4

31.e [Sister with bypass surgery prior to age of 65; sedentary; HDL <40 $mg \cdot dl^{-1}$; see table 1.1.]

32.b [Three risk factors, also age; see table 1.1.]

33.d [See table 2.1.]

34.c [ACSM recommends higher repetition range for the elderly.]

35.c [220 – age is a rough estimate, especially in the elderly.]

36.a [Estimate HRmax as 220 – age; multiply by factor in table 3.1.]

37.b [Target HR = (fractional intensity)(HRmax – HRrest) + HRrest.]

38.c [Low impact for moderate to severe arthritis.]

39.a [Target $\dot{V}O_2$ = (fractional intensity)($\dot{V}O_2$max − 3.5) + 3.5; calculate body mass in kg as lb / 2.2; solve for workload in the following equation: $\dot{V}O_2$ for arm cycling = 3.5 + 3(work-rate) / (body mass); calculate power in W as workload in kg · m · min^{-1} divided by 6.]

40.a [See table 3.1.]

Case Study A.5

41.d [Sedentary, cigarette smoker, obesity based on BMI, hypertension, LDL cholesterol >130 mg · dl^{-1}; see table 1.1.]

42.b [Calculate BMI as lb × 703 / in^2.]

43.c [Cardiac disease; see table 1.1.]

44.b [Calculate speed in m · min^{-1} as mph × 26.8; $\dot{V}O_2$ during walking = 3.5 + 0.1(speed) + 1.8(speed)(fractional grade).]

45.c [Calculate body mass in kg as lb / 2.2; convert $\dot{V}O_2$ in ml · min^{-1} · kg^{-1} to L · min^{-1}; multiply $\dot{V}O_2$ in L · min^{-1} by 5 to attain kcal · min^{-1}.]

46.b [Estimate HRmax as 220 − age, because stress test did not go to maximum; target HR − (fractional intensity)(HRmax − HRrest) + HRrest.]

47.c [Multiply estimated HRmax by factor in table 3.1.]

48.a [ACSM recommends the 10-15 rep range for cardiac patients.]

49.c [In some cases, phase II programs are reduced in length for low-risk clients, or as a result of insurance reimbursement; however, the standard length has been 12 weeks.]

50.d [Cardiovascular testing of high-risk clients must be supervised by a physician; see table 1.1.]

Case Study A.6

51.b [Sedentary, LDL cholesterol >130 mg · dl^{-1}; see table 1.1.]

52.b [Calculate BMI as lb × 703 / in^2.]

53.c [See table 1.2.]

54.b [Use reported HRmax; target HR = (fractional intensity)(HRmax – HRrest) + HRrest.]

55.c [Calculate speed in m · min^{-1} as mph × 26.8; $\dot{V}O_2$ during walking = 3.5 + 0.1(speed) + 1.8(speed)(fractional grade).]

56.a [Calculate body mass in kg as lb / 2.2; convert $\dot{V}O_2$max in ml · min^{-1} · kg^{-1} to L · min^{-1}; multiply $\dot{V}O_2$ in L · min^{-1} by 5 to attain kcal · min^{-1}.]

57.b [Target $\dot{V}O_2$ = (fractional intensity)($\dot{V}O_2$max – 3.5) + 3.5; calculate bench height in m as in. × 0.0254; solve for stepping rate using the following equation: $\dot{V}O_2$ during stepping = 3.5 + 0.2(stepping rate) + 2.4(stepping rate)(step height).]

58.b [Target $\dot{V}O_2$ = (fractional intensity)($\dot{V}O_2$max – 3.5) + 3.5; calculate body mass in kg as lb / 2.2; solve for workload in the following equation: $\dot{V}O_2$ during leg cycling = 7 + 1.8(workrate) / (body mass); calculate power in W as workload in kg · m · min^{-1} divided by 6.]

59.c [This delay is needed for surgical recovery.]

60.b [See table 2.1.]

Case Study A.7

61.c [Metabolic disease; see table 1.1.]

62.b [See Steps to Avoid Hypoglycemia.]

63.b [See table 2.1.]

64.b [See table 2.1.]

65.d [Target $\dot{V}O_2$ = (fractional intensity)($\dot{V}O_2$max – 3.5) + 3.5; select appropriate equations from page 50.]

66.d [Estimate HRmax as 220 – age; target HR = (fractional intensity)(HRmax – HRrest) + HRrest.]

67.c [See table 9.1.]

68.d [See table 9.1.]

69.b [See Steps to Avoid Hypoglycemia.]

70.a [See table 2.1.]

Case Study A.8

71.d [Calculate BMI as lb × 703 / in² or kg / height in meters²; see table 1.2.]

72.a [Enter current height and desired BMI into BMI equation and solve for weight.]

73.a [Low end of ACSM intensity range is used for those with type 2 diabetes and those needing weight loss.]

74.d [Duration and frequency need to be high to maximize caloric expenditure.]

75.c [Use known HRmax; target HR = (fractional intensity)(HRmax − HRrest) + HRrest.]

76.b [Target $\dot{V}O_2$ = (fractional intensity)($\dot{V}O_2$max − 3.5) + 3.5; solve for walking speed in the following equation: $\dot{V}O_2$ during walking = 3.5 + 0.1(speed) + 1.8(speed)(fractional grade); *Note:* Because the grade is zero, the last term drops out; calculate speed in mph as m · min⁻¹ divided by 26.8.]

77.c [Calculate body mass in kg as lb / 2.2; net $\dot{V}O_2$ = gross $\dot{V}O_2$ − 3.5; convert $\dot{V}O_2$ in ml · min⁻¹ · kg⁻¹ to L · min⁻¹; multiply $\dot{V}O_2$ in L · min⁻¹ by 5 to attain kcal · min⁻¹; because 1 lb of fat contains 3,500 kcal, divide this value by the net caloric expenditure rate to obtain total minutes needed, and then convert to hours.]

78.a [See table 9.1.]

79.b [See Steps to Avoid Hypoglycemia.]

80.c [Exercise training improves insulin sensitivity, and patients may need to reduce hypoglycemic medications.]

Case Study A.9

81.a [See table 1.1; BMI of 29.2 kg · m⁻² is "overweight," but not obese.]

82.c [PAD is a form of cardiovascular disease; see table 1.1.]

83.c [PAD reduces the systolic blood pressure measured at the ankle.]

84.a [PAD patients need to exercise the affected region.]

85.c [Continued aerobic exercise provides central cardiovascular adaptations.]

86.c [PAD patients should exercise at the highest tolerable level to achieve improvements; see the claudication scale in chapter 10]

87.b [Calculate workload in kg · m · min^{-1} as W multiplied by 6; calculate body mass in kg as lb / 2.2; $\dot{V}O_2$ during leg cycling $= 7 + 1.8$(workrate) / (body mass).]

88.a [Net $\dot{V}O_2 =$ gross $\dot{V}O_2 - 3.5$; convert net $\dot{V}O_2$ in ml · min^{-1} · kg^{-1} to L · min^{-1}; multiply $\dot{V}O_2$ in L · min^{-1} by 5 to attain kcal · min^{-1}.]

89.a [Target $\dot{V}O_2 =$ (fractional intensity)($\dot{V}O_2 - 3.5$) $+ 3.5$; solve for workload in the following equation: $\dot{V}O_2$ during leg cycling $= 7 + 1.8$(workrate) / (body mass); calculate power in W as workload in kg · m · min^{-1} divided by 6; *Note:* The answer is somewhat less than 50% of maximal power because of the component for unloaded cycling in the $\dot{V}O_2$ equation.]

90.d [Beta-blockers reduce cardiac stimulation, thus reducing HR; also, some beta-blockers have intrinsic *a*-adrenergic properties, which can result in peripheral vasoconstriction and thus decrease time to claudication.]

Case Study A.10

91.a [Women who were not exercising prior to pregnancy should seek physician clearance to exercise.]

92.d [Supine exercise is contraindicated after the first trimester.]

93.a [Excessive heat may interfere with the closure of the neural tube during the first trimester.]

94.d [Exercise during pregnancy is generally safe for mother and fetus; one benign side effect is slightly lower birth weight.]

95. b [There is little value in performing maximal exercise tests during pregnancy.]

96. b [Cardiovascular changes during pregnancy reduce the usefulness of HR and $\dot{V}O_2$ prescriptions.]

97. c [Exercise can be gradually increased throughout postpartum but generally will not reach prepregnancy levels until four to six weeks postpartum.]

98. d [Exercise during pregnancy has many positive effects.]

99. a [HRmax decreases and HRrest increases during pregnancy.]

100. c [Exercise may continue during the third trimester; non-weight-bearing exercises may become easier and safer to perform.]

Index

Note: The italicized *f* and *t* following page numbers refer to figures and tables, respectively.

About the Authors

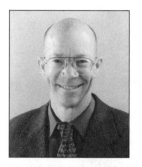

David P. Swain, PhD, has been an exercise science researcher and educator for more than 20 years. He is a professor of exercise physiology at Old Dominion University. Dr. Swain is a certified Exercise Specialist and Program Director for the ACSM and is also a Certified Strength and Conditioning Specialist of the National Strength and Conditioning Association. The ACSM named him a Fellow in 1986. Dr. Swain authored the key research studies that established the use of $\dot{V}O_2$ reserve for exercise prescription, which has been adopted by the ACSM. He is the editor of the Exercise Prescription section of the upcoming sixth edition of the *ACSM's Resource Manual for Guidelines for Exercise Testing and Prescription.*

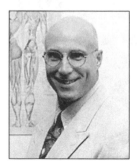

Brian C. Leutholtz, PhD, is a professor of exercise physiology at Baylor University, where he specializes in exercise prescription for special populations and also sports nutrition. Dr. Leutholtz is a Fellow of and certified Program Director for the ACSM.